LECITHIN
AND HEALTH

FRANK ORTHOEFER
Ph.D.

Lecithin and Health

by Frank T. Orthoefer, Ph.D.

Orthoefer, Frank T., 1941–
      Lecithin and health / Frank Orthoefer. — 1st ed.
      p. cm.
      Includes bibliographical references and index.
      ISBN: 1-890612-03-0

      1. Lecithin—Therapeutic use. I. Title.

RM666.L4078 1998   631.2'8
                          QBI98-355

Printed in the United States of America by United Graphics, Inc., Mattoon, IL.

Design by Studio 2D, Champaign, IL.

Cover photo by David Richard

Vital Health Publishing
P.O. Box 544
Bloomingdale, IL 60108

CONTENTS

ABOUT THE AUTHOR: Frank Orthoefer has been actively involved in lecithin research and development for more than 25 years. He has published extensively with more than 100 papers in scientific journals, texts and reference books and holds several patents (17). He has presented numerous papers at scientific meetings on his work on lecithin production, uses and nutrition. He holds BS and MS degrees from the Ohio State University, a PhD in Food Technology from Michigan State University and an MBA from the University of Illinois.

PREFACE

The U.S. population is aging. Over the past 96 years in the U.S., life expectancy increased from 47.3 years in 1900, to 74.1 years in 1981 and to age 76 in 1996. From 1960 to 1994, the population 85 years and over grew by 274%. As we collectively grow older, we become more concerned about our own health, evaluating our nutritional status and learning how nutrition affects our longevity. The thousands of books, pamphlets and commercials that continually bombard us promote various products and theories of what is "good for you." Each one attempts to provide a product, an ingredient, a supplement or an alternative therapy that will satisfy a health need, help a medical problem, or guide us toward a long and healthy life. We, as consumers, are also continually looking for a product that will slow aging, cure an illness, prevent a disease or promote wellness. Through all the scientific and popular journals and articles, there is one such substance that has not been mentioned often enough nor has it been the subject of many promotions. That substance is *lecithin*. Those people who are already familiar with health foods and nutrition may be knowledgeable of lecithin, but for the most part it is a little-known essential nutrient that is basic to all aspects of life. Consequently, lecithin is an important nutrient for us to include in our daily diets.

Lecithin's use as a nutrient and as a supplement has been reported to be an aid for various illnesses ranging from curing cardiovascular disease to improving mental function. Lecithin is widely utilized in almost all food preparations and many cosmetics as a mixing or blending agent (emulsifier). In this crucial function, it acts to promote the mixing of oil with water. Health food stores, some pharmacies and drug stores are the only places that carry lecithin on their shelves in various pure forms that range from liquids to powders, granules to encapsulated forms. All are intended for oral consumption. We have known about lecithin for years, but little has been understood about its function, metabolism, and critical physiological role in our bodies. As research continues and we discover the many important roles of lecithin in our bodily functions, it expands in importance from its role as a simple emulsifier to a more important role as a vital nutrient. It is now possible to describe this growing role based on the recent cellular research and molecular biology studies being done on lecithin. This research has significant implications toward our health. We should all know more about lecithin as a nutrient and its importance as a supplement to our diet. Its role is essential. The topics that will be discussed in this book include some technical definitions of lecithin terminology; food sources of lecithin; how lecithin is made or isolated; its properties, uses and biochemistry; its effects on our body; how lecithin affects our health; and some recipes for lecithin as an addition to foods.

You are invited to read through this discussion of the latest scientific findings. It is my aim to provide you, the health conscious consumer, with greater insight into this natural substance and to describe its properties and characteristics. Once you are aware of what lecithin is, its role in your biochemistry and nutritional status, and its importance to health, you will want to make lecithin a part of your daily diet. It may well be the miracle nutrient that serves as your pathway to optimum health.

CHAPTER 1

Description of Lecithin

1.1 The Importance and Source of Lecithin

The term "lecithin" refers not to a single, natural compound, but to a class of compounds. It is found in every living cell, whether it is of plant or animal origin. Biochemists tell us that it is involved in *all* processes of life: breathing, metabolism, energy production and transport, and nerve function. Lecithin is a fat-like compound present in cell structures, which participates in metabolism, and is a source of essential nutrients. It has been discovered to have vital health benefits for:

- Normalizing reproductive health,
- Enhancing liver and heart health,
- Improving memory,
- Increasing physical performance,
- Lowering risks of cancer.

Even the term "lecithin" implies importance, having been derived from the Greek "Lekithos," meaning egg yolk. The egg is the symbol of birth, life, fertility, strength, and comfort. Lecithin was first discovered in egg yolk. Approximately ten percent of a fresh yolk is lecithin. Egg yolk once was the raw material for the commercial isolation of lecithin, but pharmaceutical companies produce today only small quantities from eggs. This highly nutritious lecithin has been used for the preparation of intravenously injectable fatty nutrient solutions for patients who no longer are able to eat a normal diet. Today, the main commercial source of lecithin, including that used in injectables, is the soybean.

Lecithin is present in many of the foods we consume, but it is most concentrated in the same foods that are high in cholesterol and fats (Table 1). Organ meats, red meats and eggs are the most *concentrated* sources of dietary lecithin. However, with the current trend in eating habits toward low-calorie and low-cholesterol diets, people are limiting their consumption of fatty foods. Because lecithin is a constituent of the foods people are avoiding, they are also unwittingly limiting

TABLE 1 *Lecithin Content of Common Foods*

Food	Lecithin (mg/serving)	Food	Lecithin (mg/serving)
Lecithin Supplement (1 tbsp granules)	1,725.00	Lecithin Supplement (1 soft gel capsule)	180.00
Egg (1 large)	3,362.55	Beef Steak (3.5 oz.)	466.12
Peanuts (1 oz.)	107.35	Cauliflower (1/2 cup)	107.06
Coffee (6 oz.)	2.05	Infant Formula (1 cup)	23.77
Orange (1 medium)	53.03	Human Milk (1 cup)	27.08
Potato (1 medium)	25.97	Milk (whole, 1 cup)	27.91
Grape Juice (6 oz.)	2.11	Iceberg Lettuce (1 oz.)	2.86
Tomato (1 medium)	4.94	Apple (1 medium)	29.87
Banana (1 medium)	3.26	Whole Wheat Bread (1 slice)	6.57
Cucumber (1/2 cup)	3.06	Butter (1 tsp.)	6.80
Ginger Ale (12 oz.)	1.11	Margarine (1 tsp.)	1.74
Corn Oil (1 tbsp.)	0.13		

their intake of lecithin[1,2]. Particularly significant is the reduction of egg consumption (20%), organ meats (50%) and red meats (48%) most likely resulting in an inadequate dietary intake of lecithin and choline, a component of lecithin. According to USDA's Economic Research Service, the average American consumed 12 fewer pounds of red meat in 1996 than 20 years ago. The average American, even with all the varied uses of lecithin, consumes only about 3g/day[3] although others have estimated the consumption at about 6g/day.[4] Other supplemental sources, over and above the normal diet, are likely required for sufficient dietary intake of lecithin. Whole soy food consumption, which is increasing annually in the U.S., may help to increase the level of lecithin consumption, but at its current levels is still far from adding significant amounts to the average diet. For cholesterol reduction, the consumption of soy products supplies not only lecithin, but fiber and protein as well, which are also known to contribute toward this end[5].

The diet of the average American also has less lecithin than that of the previous generation because more purified and refined foods are being developed to facilitate today's food distribution system. In addition, consumer's have expressed demands for faster food preparation and a general preference for prepared foods with a bland taste. With the current demand for low-fat, low-calorie foods, a further decrease in consumption of lecithin is occurring, possibly even to the point where consumption is at sub-optimum levels for health. With the reduction in lecithin consumption, there is obviously a decreased intake of its components such as a bioavailable source of choline, itself an essential nutrient.

Of course, many people, including those doing research on this nutrient, are aware of the nutritional attributes of lecithin. They are convinced of the positive results brought about by adding lecithin to their diets. Health food consumers are often able to recite the "lore" of lecithin with attributes such as: "cleans your arteries, renews your energy, keeps you youthful, enhances your health and improves your learning"[3,6,7]. These are powerful claims to be made for a little known, commonly found food ingredient. One would think that lecithin is a nutrient that can make a "new you." Although it may not be considered a "fountain of youth," it certainly is a nutrient that contributes to well-being[8]. The most recent scientific evidence is convincing. Lecithin is important in your diet.

1.2 *An Overview*

Our eating habits have evolved over the years through various phases and fads: high-protein diets, low-calorie diets, vegetarian diets and carbohydrate diets. Our perspective has evolved to the USDA's expression of the new food pyramid. We count calories, avoid fats, add polyunsaturated fats and omega 3 fatty acids, eat more fruits and vegetables, take vitamins, minerals and other supplemental aids. We even exercise more. All of these things are an attempt to attain a better physical, biochemical and nutritional state. All of us are searching for a path leading to better health. If we just had one miracle nutrient or a combination of supplements that would allow us to live longer and be healthier, it would be especially beneficial and highly prized. Of course, this miracle nutrient as a single entity is unknown. Nutritional sciences have progressed beyond the single essential "vitamin" concept to embracing an entire spectrum of nutrients that contribute to general well being.

We have learned much about nutrition and are continually updating our knowledge of new nutrients and supplements to take for our general health. Even non-nutrients have been found to have a role. Most of us now know of the importance of dietary fiber and the consequences of consuming more refined foods. By not getting sufficient fiber in our diets, we have subjected ourselves to a higher likelihood of diverticulitis, colon cancer, cardiovascular problems and even a higher incidence of diabetes. We accept the importance of fiber in our diets and we are finding more products on the grocery shelves like high fiber breads, cereals, and whole grains that add back what the refined foods have taken away.

Statistically, the fact is that we are living longer, but that doesn't mean we are necessarily healthier. We have conquered many safety issues in food processing and have learned how to treat many diseases. Yet the cost of healthcare continues to rise by leaps and bounds. Pharmaceutical suppliers are selling more drugs than ever. These drugs, even though amazing and necessary, have side effects, some of which may be severe and even catastrophic. And none of them is a miracle cure. Many people are taking cholesterol-reducing drugs. Yet by-pass surgeries are common place. Vascular disease, circulatory problems and gallstones are common. In addition, as we grow older, we see an increased incidence of memory loss, forgetfulness and Alzheimer's disease. Nursing homes are commonly used to care for people with these problems. We take new drugs, obscure nutrients, new food additives, non-caloric synthetic fats and bioengineered lipids, all in hopes of improving our diet and general well being. Similar to the dietary fiber story, sometimes we forget the more natural solution.

There are a vast number of food products on the market today that have been formulated for widespread appeal to the consumer, many with little or no attention to nutrition. These foods meet the needs for convenience in preparation, general taste appeal, fast food markets or microwave preparation. With our busy lifestyles, it is easier to grab these foods as we are "on the run." Some activists have used the terms "plastic" and/or "junk" foods to describe the character of these formulated foods.

I believe, as do other food and nutritional biochemists, that we are still missing some vital nutrients in many of the foods listed on today's menus. Nutrients that had been in our forebearers' diets have been partially or completely eliminated from the current food supply due to the requirement of the food industry for shorter processing ease, extended shelf life, and consumer convenience.

Before WWII, diets were less purified than ours today. However, little was known about the negative health effects of eating high-fat diets, and so we consumed large amounts of organ meats, red meats, whole eggs, whole milk with cream, dairy cream and liver. All of these foods, eaten in large quantities, are considered unhealthy today. However, prior to this shift in thinking, we also consumed an abundance of unrefined vegetable oils and more whole grains and cereals. Surprisingly the diets of old were, in some ways, more nutritional, but extremely high in calories and fat. Those excess calories with a high fat content are definitely ill-advised, especially with today's more sedentary lifestyles.

As the safety of our food supply evolved, and with the recognition of the importance of multivitamins, mineral fortification, low-fat diets, more fruits, vegetables and whole grains, what could possibly be missing that affects our general well being? What could increase our energy, help speed the transport of essential nutrients to the vital organs of our body, quicken our cellular responses and assist in the neurotransmission of our brain and nervous cells? Surprisingly, there is a single class of compounds that was present in all those foods that we no longer consume in large amounts: organ meats, red meats, whole eggs, dairy cream and liver. This forgotten nutrient is called *lecithin*. It has come to the forefront of nutritional awareness and is being scientifically investigated by well-known nutritional biochemists worldwide. I believe, after you have read this book, you will want to include lecithin in your daily diet.

1.3 *A Word of Caution*

Many nutritionists, biochemists and physicians, as well as individuals interested in promoting optimum health, have published articles on the benefits of food fortification. Sometimes, the particular nutrients are referred to as supplements, alternative or complementary therapies, functional foods or even "health foods." Unfortunately, some of the information used in making these claims has been based on anecdotal (interpreted) evidence and not necessarily scientifically derived data. Much of the earlier information available on lecithin has been based on anecdotal evidence. Some, myself included, have called lecithin a "miracle food" based on my own personal experience. While anecdotal reports are true to the observer, and may be somewhat valuable for further study, many are not valid. Observations may be incorrectly associated with "cause and effect." Anecdotal information can be misleading as well. For example, if you read something often enough or if a supposed authority tells you often enough, you will likely believe it. The "spin doctors" in political campaigns are experts at this. Further, even in the most highly controlled studies, the false pill or placebo effect is well known to influence the outcome of clinical trials. A positive effect is seen just because the study is being conducted. Actual correlation to good health may be misinterpreted. Proper statistics are required to show if an effect is real. We have to remember that "figures don't lie" and "good science has no substitute."

This short book is presented as an easily understood summary on the attributes and importance of lecithin to good health. The scientific literature covering this single class of compounds is much more extensive than the average consumer possibly imagines. I have attempted to be objective in summarizing the science. Sometimes, however, even the literature is contradictory and disagreements are not uncommon. This book is not exhaustive, either in a review of the literature or in a technical sense. What I have relied upon are the results of controlled scientific investigations that have been subjected to statistical evaluation and peer review. I also rely on a limited number of anecdotal quotes, but only for emphasis. Even with this limitation of using only statistically accurate information on lecithin, startling results on prevention and cures have been found and will be discussed. I believe it will help you to see the value and importance of lecithin. You will be able to judge whether or not it is a critically valuable nutrient to be added to your diet based on the efforts of many nutritionists, biochemists, and medical professionals in defining the role of lecithin.

1.4 *Definitions and Structures of Lecithin*

There is no simple definition of lecithin since it is a class of compounds. In scientific literature you can find references that call lecithin "phosphatidylcholine." Other synonyms used for lecithin are phospholipids, phosphatides, (k)cephalins and even sphingomyelins. It is little wonder that studying lecithin can lead to confusion[9]. Sometimes you find the word "lecithin" being used just for the definition of an oil-free powdered product. This interchange of terminology leads to confusion by investigators, researchers, medical practitioners, consumers and all others concerned with lecithin and its benefits. Chemists and even science writers often use all three terms (phosphatidylcholine, lecithin and phospholipids) interchangeably when discussing lecithin, leading to yet more confusion. The term "lecithin" actually designates commercial products, but may also refer to a particular chemical composition at the same time. For our purposes, "lecithin" will be used to define the natural mixture of various phospholipids found in commercial soybean-derived products. Phospholipids will refer to those substances that possess a structure similar to fat but have phosphorous in the molecule. Remember that the term lecithin refers to a compound or a mixture of components. Pure "lecithins" will be designated as phosphatidylcholine or phosphatidylserine, for example.

Chemically, phospholipids (phosphatides) include all lipoidal compounds, which contain phosphorous in their molecules (Figure 1). The chemical structure of lecithin is surprisingly similar to that of the food oils (e.g. soybean oil, corn oil, cottonseed oil, olive oil, peanut oil, and sunflower oil). The phospholipids are essential components and are found in every plant and animal cell. The phosphate group in the molecule is the common chemical structure of all lecithins. The phospholipids have been divided into 1) lecithins 2) cephalins, and 3) sphingomyelins. When completely hydrolyzed or broken down, each molecule of a lecithin will yield two molecules of fatty acid, one molecule each of glycerol, phosphoric acid, and a nitrogenous or other base compound (usually choline). The fatty acids present are usually linoleic acid, linolenic acid,

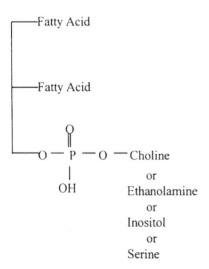

Figure 1. Chemical Species Referred to as Lecithin

oleic acid, palmitic acid and stearic aid. Choline, the nitrogen-containing base, is classed as a member of the B complex vitamins. Its function in the body is to prevent accumulation of fat in the liver and in the transmission of nerve impulses across cholinergic synapses. (Figure 2). The representations may be in the a lecithin and b lecithin forms. The naturally occurring lecithin is the a lecithin and is represented below where R_1 and R_2 represent different fatty acids:

$$CH_2OOCR_1$$

$$CHOOCR_2$$

$$CH_2OPOCH_2CH_2N(CH_3)^3$$

Lecithin is a mixture of phospholipids (phosphatides) that may be divided into:

I. Phosphatidylcholine (lecithin)

    a. fatty acids

        1. linoleic acid

        2. palmitic acid

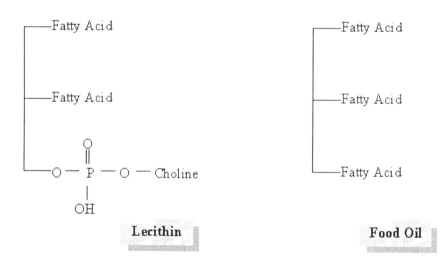

Figure 2. Comparison of Lecithin and Food Oil (triglyceride) Structure

3. stearic acid

4. oleic acid

b. glycerol

c. phosphoric acid

d. choline

II. Cephalins

a. phosphatidylethanolamine

b. phosphatidylinositol

c. phosphatidylserine

III. Sphingomyelins

a. Fatty acids

b. phosphoric acid

c. choline

d. sphingosine—unsaturated amino alcohol

In the strictest chemical definition, only phosphatidylcholine is "lecithin." (K)Cephalin is the term used for phosphatidylserine and phosphatidyl ethanolamine. Phospholipids and phosphatides refer to the whole group. The common phospholipids, as with fats and oils, are structured about a glycerol backbone:

CH_2OH

$CHOH$

CH_2OH

Even with all this confusion in the definition of lecithin, we can agree that its components are varied in content and in amount, depending on its source. Some of these components, such as choline, inositol and linoleic acid, are critical to life and well being.

1.5 *The Major (and most important) Components of Lecithin for Human Health*

The components that make up lecithin are *essential* in human metabolic processes in all cells even down to the molecular level. Cell biosynthesis of lecithin does not proceed blindly and automatically, but it is dependent upon supply and need as expressed through various feedback control mechanisms. The most important components within lecithin, besides that of the *phospholipid* molecule itself, are *linoleic acid*, *choline*, and *inositol*. They effect the metabolic processes in the following ways:

1.5a Linoleic Acid

Linoleic acid, a polyunsaturated fatty acid that makes up about 60% of the fatty acids in lecithin, is present on the middle or second carbon of the glycerol "backbone" of lecithin. At this position, the linoleic acid is in a particularly active position that favors both the enzymatic activity of phospholipase A and the lecithin cholesterol acyl transferase (LCAT) enzyme system.

The amount of linoleic acid required as an essential fatty acid is apparently variable as found in studies on patients that are fed totally by injection. For parenteral nutrition where all nutrients are supplied through injectable solutions, 0.05 gm to 0.1gm/Kg body weight is needed[10]. For active individuals, without this limitation, a much larger amount of linoleic acid is most likely required.

A deficiency of linoleic acid has been described as causing changes to the skin, disturbed water balance, atrophy of reproductive glands, and the decrease or cessation of lactation. Linoleic acid deficiency can even be observed, using an electron microscope, as structural changes to the mitochondria. Restoration of a linoleic acid deficiency requires several weeks' administration of adequate amounts of linoleic acid primarily through dietary supplements using linoleic acid rich oils. Unfortunately, many of our food oils that are high in linoleic acid are readily oxidized, soybean and corn oil being among these. Lecithin, even though it is high in linoleic acid, is remarkably stable to autoxidation. I have personally stored lecithin for many years before notice-able oxidation occurs whereas vegetable oils are highly oxidized after even only a few months storage.

The physiological effects of linoleic acid as present in lecithin also are greater than that of other lipids. Linoleic acid is particularly active in lowering serum cholesterol. Several hypotheses have been presented concerning why this occurs[11]. These include:

1. Increased biological degradation of cholesterol and, therefore, in-creased excretion.

2. Removal of cholesterol from the blood and deposition in the liver through enhanced cholesterol receptor activity.

3. The solubility of cholesterol in fats decreases with an increase in iodine value. The iodine value of butter is 40 while the value for soybean oil that is high in linoleic acid is 125-130.

A simple, straightforward addition of high linoleic acid-containing leci-thin to the diet, even at moderate quantities, is recommended. This insures an adequate dietary supply of linoleic acid that is metaboli-cally active in an oxidatively stable form. It is suggested to consume two tablespoonfuls of lecithin daily, if for no other reason than as a source of linoleic acid.

1.5b Choline

The biochemical properties of choline can influence the vitality of the brain and general body behavior. Choline is required by the brain for the production of acetylcholine, a vital compound necessary for the transmission of neural messages from one nerve cell to another. Bio-chemically, choline is a methyl donor in hormone synthesis, is a con-tributor to essential amino acid and phospholipid synthesis, and is important for the circulation of fatty acids, lipids, and cholesterol[8]. Choline can be and is synthesized in the body. Logistically, the synthe-sis depends on the presence of an adequate supply of the building blocks required for synthesis. Adequate amounts of the B vitamins, folic acid and B12, along with methionine are required for the synthe-

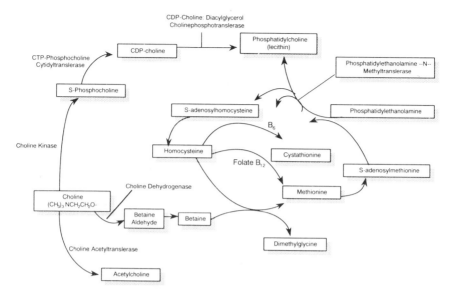

Figure 3. Choline Metabolism

sis of choline. The pathway for choline synthesis is shown in Figure 3. A biological choline deficiency will result in kidney damage, fatty liver and retarded growth. The human requirement for choline has been determined to be 1.5gm to 3gm per day.

Choline is but one of several biochemical methyl donors such as betaine and methionine. Methionine is an essential amino acid. Acceptors of the methyl group from choline are aminoethanol, homocysteine and glycine. Physiologically, choline affects lipid transport from the liver. It is quite likely the choline effect on lipid transport occurs through its affect on lecithin synthesis. Choline apparently promotes lecithin synthesis. Research has recently shown that high levels of homocysteine, a sulfur-containing amino acid that is also a methyl group acceptor, increases the risk of CVD (heart attack) (30%), strokes (31%) and myocardial infarction (32%)[30,31,33]. Insufficient choline may result in increased homocysteine levels.

Acetylcholine, as a neurotransmitter, is the messenger between the brain, nerves, and organs. Acetylcholine may also be involved in a wide range of other normal brain activities that includes learning, memory, sensation, motor coordination, and sleep, as well as the bodily functions of respiration, circulation and digestion. Acetylcholine is split or hydrolyzed by the enzyme, cholinesterase, in a very rapid reaction lasting about two thousandths of a second. This splitting reaction is constantly and uniformly repeated at all the thousands of nerve cell synapses. If one disrupts the cholinesterase reaction, it is fatal. Nerve gases and extreme toxins are examples of inhibitors of cholinesterase.

The most important sources in the body for the formation of acetylcholine are lecithin and choline. Ingestion of free choline, however, is less effective than ingestion of phosphatidylcholine. Consequently, phosphatidylcholine is the preferred dietary component. Over 99% of the choline present in the diet is in the form of lecithin or phosphatidylcholine[8]. In granular or de-oiled lecithin, phosphatidylcholine makes up about 23% of the mixture. In a liquid lecithin supplement, it is only about 15%. One tablespoon of granular lecithin provides about 1725 mg-phosphatidylcholine and 232 mg choline. One capsule of a liquid lecithin supplement contains about 180 mg of phosphatidylcholine and 24mg of choline, not nearly as concentrated as the granular form. Free choline, when consumed as an alternative to phosphatidylcholine, is rapidly degraded by bacteria in the intestine forming trimethylamine, which is a fishy-odored degradation product. Pure lecithin ingestion does not give a fishy odor.

Choline is a component of plasmalogen, a phospholipid found at high levels in heart muscle cell membranes. Acute myocardial ischemia (coronary arterial disease) may be the result of plasmalogen breakdown[15]. The breakdown of plasmalogen occurs through activation of the enzyme PLA-2 phospholipase. Disruption of membrane permeability and ion transport also causes abnormal heart contractions.

The choline component of phosphatidylcholine is an essential nutrient in many animal species, including man. Choline deficiency causes the development of fatty liver, an initial stage that may result in more severe liver disease. Choline deficiency also leads to abnormal kidney function, infertility, impaired growth, bone abnormalities, decreased hematopoiesis (synthesis of red blood cells) and hypertension[4]. Other lecithin or phospholipid components do not have the essential characteristic of the choline present in phosphatidylcholine. Other more common sources than lecithin of ethanolamine, inositol or serine are present in the diet. Even so, phosphatidylserine or one of the other phospholipids may also be a dietary component contributing to good health. Phosphatidylserine will be discussed in Chapters 2 & 5.

1.5c Inositol

Inositol, another component of lecithin, is found in many green plants, muscle tissue and cereal grains. In most cases, it is present as the hexaphosphate derivative that is also called phytic acid. In humans, inositol is present in highest quantities in the microsomes of the liver, kidney, spleen, in all cell fractions of the brain, and in high concentration in the lens of the eye.

A deficiency of inositol results in stunting of growth, alopecia (loss of hair), and fatty degeneration of the liver. Inositol, in the form of the hexaphosphate or phytic acid, affects the availability of iron, zinc and calcium. Vitamin D suppresses the phytic acid effect on mineral availability. There are no known inositol deficiency diseases because of its widespread distribution in foods.

1.6 *Properties of Lecithin.*

While lecithin is not a vitamin, it contains significant amounts of choline and inositol, which are classified as vitamins. While it is similar to a vegetable oil, being a rich source of polyunsaturated fatty acids, it is not classified as an oil. It is not a mineral, but it contains a generous portion of organic phosphorous. Rather, lecithin is a complex mixture of all these substances. The benefits of taking lecithin are sound and the biochemical attributes are proven, particularly as seen with the importance of phosphatidylcholine, phosphatidylserine, linoleic acid and inositol. Lecithin in its purest state looks and feels like a waxy solid. In de-oiled or oil-free forms, it is produced as granules or powder. In vegetable oil solutions, even at high concentrations, it appears as a very thick oil. Lecithin is not water soluble but will hydrate to a thick gel depending on the concentration. Lecithin hydrates are generally opaque white to light yellow in color.

1.7 *Where Lecithin is Found*

Lecithin is found in the main reproductive or propagative tissues of plants such as seeds, nuts, and grains. It is also found in egg yolks, organ tissues and other meats. The lecithin available from the pharmacy or health food store for use as a supplement is extracted from soybeans[9]. In terms of current research, it is one of the many substances from soybeans being investigated for potential benefits in lowering the risk of cardiovascular disease (CVD) and cancer[5]. In our bodies as well as that of animals, lecithin is concentrated in the vital organs (brain, liver, and kidneys). Within the individual cell, the lecithin is contained in the outer cell membrane. Here, lecithin directs the flow of nutrients, hormones, and waste products into and out of the cell. Communication within the cell, as well as with other cells, is controlled by lecithin. Sophisticated structures called micelles, bilayer sheets, and liposomes are all structures of the cell that depend upon the unique physical properties of lecithin and its behavior as a nutrient.

1.8 *Commercial Lecithin and Its Composition*

Commercial lecithin for use as a food ingredient, a nutritional supplement, a functional food or a health food may be isolated from sunflower, canola, rapeseed, corn or soybeans[9,16]. Most is from soybeans. Soybeans, the richest source, contain 0.5% to 1.0% lecithin (Table 2). Approximately 100 Kg (220 lbs.) of soybeans are required to produce 200 gm (approx. ½ lb.) of lecithin.

The lecithin purchased at the health food store or pharmacy as a liquid or in gelatin capsules is a natural mix of components rather than a single chemical entity. This lecithin is recovered from extracted soybean oil by simply adding water to the oil, separating the hydrated

TABLE 2 *Composition of Soybeans*

Item	Range	Item	Range
Protein	35%–42%	Fat	18%–20%
Lecithin	0.5%–1.5%	CH_2O	24%–26%
Fiber	4%–6%	Minerals	4%–5%
Water	10%–12%		

TABLE 3 *Composition of Crude Lecithin from Soybean Oil*

Item	Range	Item	Range
Lecithin	60%–70%	Soybean Oil	30%–35%
Water	<1%	Other* Phospholipids	<1%

*Other phospholipids consist of cardiolipids, phosphatidylglycerol, lysolecithin and phosphatidic acid.

lecithin, and drying. The lecithin, often referred to as "crude lecithin," at that point is a viscous, dark and wax-like material (Table 3). Minor additions of vegetable oil and free fatty acids from vegetable oil liquefy or fluidize the waxy lecithin. This fluid lecithin may then be used in capsule production or may be sold as liquid lecithin for use in food formulations. Highly concentrated dry, granular lecithin as well as powders are also produced. These are made from the crude lecithin by nearly complete removal of the oil from the wax-like crude lecithin[8]. Fractionation of the crude lecithin into the various purified components such as phosphatidylcholine or phosphatidylserine is performed by chromatography. The benefit of the higher concentration of phospholipids in granular lecithin is easily seen as higher potency. A new lecithin tablet without gelatin or dispersants was recently made available that is 98% active compared to the 50% activity in capsules.

Waxlike soybean lecithin contains other minor phospholipids plus other substances such as:

- cardiolipids

- phosphoglycerol

- lysolecithin (minus a fatty acid)

- phosphatidic acid[9]

These substances are not known to have particular health benefits. The average composition of soybean lecithin is shown in Table 4. The fatty acid and mineral composition is shown in Table 5. Lecithin is also a source of polyunsaturated fatty acids. About 60% of the fatty acids present are linoleic acid, an essential fatty acid.

TABLE 4 *Average Composition of Soybean Lecithin in Liquid and Granular Forms*

Molecule	Liquid	Granules or Powder
Phospholipids	65%	98%
Phosphatidylcholine	15%	23%
Phosphatidylethanolamine	14%	21%
Phosphatidylinositol	13%	19%
Other Phospholipids	10%	15%
Phosphatidic Acid	4%	6%
Glycolipids	9%	14%
Other Components	35%	2%

TABLE 5 *Fatty Acid and Mineral Composition of Soybean Lecithin*

Fatty Acids	Liquid	Granules
Palmitic Acid (16:0)	15.6%	20.3%
Stearic Acid (18:0)	4.7%	4.7%
Total Saturated	**20.3%**	**24.9%**
Oleic Acid	17.9%	9.2%
Linoleic Acid	54.0%	58.9%
Linolenic Acid	6.7%	7.0%
Total Unsaturated	**78.6%**	**75.1%**
Phosphorous	2.0%	3.0%
K (potassium)	0.44%	0.8%
Ca (calcium)	0.04%	0.07%
Mg (magnesium)	0.06%	0.09%
Na (sodium)	0.01%	0.03%

CHAPTER 2

Lecithin Biology (How it Works)

2.1 Introduction

Lecithin, when consumed and assimilated as a part of the diet, is a source of unsaturated fatty acids as well as the essential vitamins, choline and inositol. As such, it has several distinct biological functions (Figure 4). When we look for lecithin in the body, we find it to be a component of all cell membranes and even subcellular structures[10,11]. It is involved in carrying the chemical messages between cells that allow them to function as a group rather than as individual cells.

2.2 Cell Membranes

Cell membranes, the outer layers that keep the cells intact and whole, are necessary for the existence of life. This layer is made up of complex structures that separate and exchange substances from the external, or outside environment, with the interior portions of the cell. These membranes are structures of all living cells. Most important for higher organisms are the structures and membranes of its nerve cells. The generation of the electrical nerve impulse, its transmission

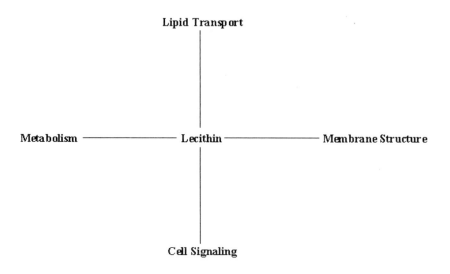

Lipid Transport

Metabolism ——————— Lecithin ——————— Membrane Structure

Cell Signaling

Figure 4. Functions of Lecithin

along the nerve cell and the relaying of the electrical impulse from one cell to another across the cell-to-cell synapse are all membrane driven. Phospholipids are an essential component of the nerve cells' membrane. The phospholipids are packed side-by-side in a double or bilayer sandwich that contains proteins, enzymes, sterols and other components (Figure 5). In animal cells, phosphatidylcholine is the most prevalent phospholipid constituent while in bacterial cells phosphatidylethanolamine is most prevalent. Other lipid-like components present are sphingomyelins and cholesterol. The membrane phospholipid content varies as shown in Table 6. The bilayers are constantly being renewed and regenerated[17]. In the liver, the half-life of a cell is one day whereas nerve and brain cells are replaced very slowly with half-lives extending for years.

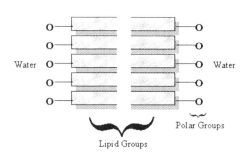

Water   Water

Polar Groups

Lipid Groups

Figure 5. Lipid Bilayer Structure
Contributing to Cell Membrane

TABLE 6 *Lipids in Cell Membranes*

Item	Choles-terol	PC	SPH	PE	PS	PI	PG	PA
Nerve sheaths	22%	11%	6%	14%	7%	(21% glycolipids)		
Red blood corpuscles in human beings	24%	23%	18%	20%	8%	3%		
Red blood corpuscles in rat	24%	31%	9%	15%	7%	2%		
Plasma membrane	24%			80%			15%	5%

Phospholipid structures also exist inside the cell. For example, the mitochondrial membranes, a subcellular structure that is the location of cell respiration, are the site for enzymes and the enzyme activity responsible for energy production. Mitochondria within the cell are composed of up to 90% phospholipids.

The membranes must be fluid (deformable) and selectively permeable. The fluidity of the phospholipid membrane depends on the ability of lecithin to behave as a liquid crystal within the bilayer[10]. It must readily change in state from a solid to a liquid crystal and back again. The shift or phase change is dependent on temperature as well as on the composition of the environment. The phase change is accompanied by a change in the permeability of the membrane as well.

2.3 *Cell Signaling*

Lecithin is the messenger that carries the signals or message from the exterior of the cell across the cell membrane to the interior of the cell where biochemical functions occur. The message may be a signal from hormones produced in other parts of the body or from many other substances exterior to the cell. "Without this process, cells could not grow, replicate, or absorb and utilize nutrients for energy"[8,10]. The outermost membrane of the cell is almost a master switch for the cell. The cell membrane controls the passage of nutrients, charged ions, molecular messages (hormones), cell-to-cell communication and even cellular shape. Proteins are embedded in the membrane and manage the activity of the cell membrane. Coordination of the activities is dependent upon the phospholipids present.

The actual first step in signaling is the activation of the "G" enzymes. The activated G enzymes then activate one or more of the several phospholipases. The phospholipases break down a specific or a targeted phospholipid into a free fatty acid plus a partial phospholipid (Figure 6). The products of phospholipid breakdown then activate protein kinase C (PKC). PKC is a central regulatory enzyme that triggers multiple reactions affecting cell growth, metabolism, nutrient uptake, ion transport, muscle contraction, and even programmed cell death

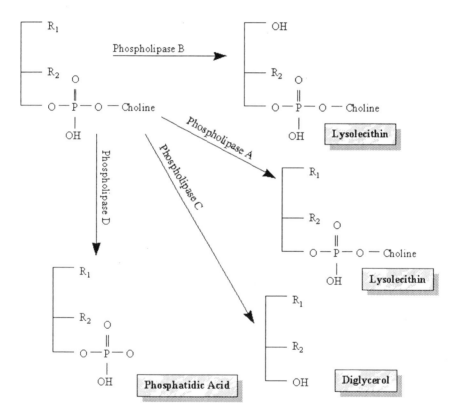

Figure 6. Enzymatic Hydrolysis of Phospholids
(R₁ and R₂ are fatty acids)

(apoptosis). Disruption or breakdown of this signaling process is thought by some to be involved in cancer and Alzheimer's disease.

Thousands upon thousands of cellular messages are generated almost simultaneously and instantaneously. The mechanism of translation into specific messages is largely unknown. Different signals apparently stimulate different G proteins, which activate the phospholipases. The different products of the phospholipase reaction also have different effects on PKC. Additionally, at least 10 different forms of PKC are known[25,26].

The coordination of cellular activity leads to a collection of cells within specific tissues or organs that perform their role as part of the total organism. Obviously, for all higher animals, including humans, all cellular systems or tissues must work in conjunction, forming various tissue or organ systems. Lecithin is involved in the signaling and coordination of cellular activity that together make up the whole organism.

2.4 *Central Nervous System and Nerve Cells*

The central nervous system contains numerous phospholipids. Phospholipids are unique in that they are one of the few compounds that pass the blood-brain barrier. Lecithin, as a source of choline, is utilized in the formation of acetylcholine, a major neurotransmitter. Acetylcholine deficiency has been associated with various nerve diseases including Alzheimer's disease or Huntington's chorea. Lecithin administration has proven highly effective in treating severe mental disorders[27]. Lecithin is unique in being readily available as a nutrient, simple to administer through the diet and an effective but harmless food supplement with no known undesirable side effects[28].

The cellular membranes of nerve cells are particularly high in phosphatidylserine. Phosphatidylserine may have the specialized function of anchoring many of the proteins in the membrane matrix. Among the membrane proteins are ATPase, kinases, and receptors. Cell-to-cell communication is believed to occur through a hydrolyzed phosphatidylserine among others. Some research scientists working in this field have postulated phosphatidylserine involvement also includes antigen stability, receptor activity and growth factors.

The cell membrane is distinctly different on the outside vs. the inside of the bilayer. Phosphatidylserine is the most noted example. Phosphatidylserine is located almost exclusively on the inner half of the bilayer or cell side of the cell membrane. Enzymes can change the position of the phosphatidylserine from the inside to the outside of the cell. When the position changes, the accumulation of phosphatidylserine on the outer side apparently signals that the cell has become old or injured and should be re-cycled. It is the immune cells that eliminate the cells with phosphatidylserine on the outer surface. This is also believed to be important for nerve cell receptor function. In animal trials, age-related receptor abnormalities were found to be partially normalized by dietary phosphatidylserine administration. Phosphatidylserine, in separate studies, was found to stimulate nerve growth factor synthesis involved in nerve tissue regeneration.

Numerous animal studies have shown phosphatidylserine to stimulate dopamine synthesis, induce dopamine release, and reverse fading EEG signals that have been correlated with diminishing memory functions. Other results have shown a reversal of growth factor receptor density and enhanced nerve growth factor production. Neither the amino acid serine nor other phospholipids were found to substitute for phosphatidylserine in many experiments.

2.5   *Lecithin Synthesis*

Various pathways are known for the synthesis of specific phospholipids. Humans can even form some of the building blocks that go into the synthesis of lecithin. Other components are derived exclusively from dietary sources. For example, choline may be derived from the amino acids methionine and cysteine. The polyunsaturated fatty acid, linoleic acid, cannot be synthesized and is essential to the diet. Other polyunsaturated fatty acids can be synthesized from dietary linoleic fatty acid. It seems rather unlikely there is an essential requirement for any specific phospholipid since the components may be derived from various metabolic pathways as well as diet. By definition, an essential nutrient is any substance that cannot be made in adequate quantities in our bodies. Lecithin does not currently qualify, although with more research it may be found to qualify. Additionally, a deficiency disease results when an essential nutrient is withheld. Recent evidence suggests lecithin to be important but likely not essential. Even though our bodies can synthesize lecithin, perhaps it is not at sufficient quantities or at the proper time or location to satisfy particular needs. Studies are currently being performed, however, to show that lecithin, particularly phosphatidylcholine, is essential for a healthy, optimal diet.

Actual lecithin synthesis occurs in several locations including the mitochondria of the cell as well as in its microsomes and endoplasmic reticulum. As readily seen, its synthesis requires the presence of many components. Among these are glycerol, phosphorous, fatty acids, choline and serine. It seems advisable from a dietary management perspective to ensure that no gaps in supply of these building blocks exist. Supplementing the food supply with this readily available nutrient seems to be "cheap" insurance. Additionally, many believe that the intake today of lecithin is insufficient and that the levels are inadequate in our food supply. They recommend the use of lecithin as a food supplement.

Phospholipid blends have been promoted and sold previously by pharmaceutical companies. One of these mixtures was made up of a modified high linoleic acid phosphatidylcholine and was used in the treatment of liver diseases and disturbed fat metabolism. Combinations with other therapeutic substances have been made for capsule preparation as well as injectable solutions. No harmful side effects are known to occur with these synthesized or special lecithin blends. The expense associated with the synthesized lecithin and specialty blends is not necessary for dietary supplementation. Naturally derived lecithin is more than adequate.

CHAPTER 3

Lecithin in Relation to Other Nutrients

3.1 *Cholesterol, Lecithin and Lipids*

There are volumes of information on the negative aspects of cholesterol in health and nutrition. It may be surprising, but the presence of cholesterol is vital to the body and its normal functions. Cholesterol is involved in the synthesis of vitamin D, sex and adrenal hormones, and bile salts. These functions are important aspects of fat metabolism. Cholesterol is a functional component of cell membranes, active in transport of nutrients and a structural component of cell walls.

The cholesterol present in the foods we eat, along with that synthesized in the liver, contribute to the total amount found in the body. Dietary cholesterol is absorbed from the foods we eat in the proximal jejunum (adjacent to the duodenum) in the form of a package called micelles. Micelles are loosely bound complexes of bile, lipids including cholesterol and degraded products from lipid hydrolysis. The cholesterol in our diet is largely free cholesterol. When absorbed, between 60 and 80% of the cholesterol from the micelles is esterified becoming cholesterol ester. This function is performed by the enzyme cholesterol esterase, a non-specific enzyme. As the ester, cholesterol is absorbed into the lymph in the form of chylomicrons and also through the very low-density lipoproteins (VLDL). The body produces far more cholesterol than is in the normal diet. All tissues are able to synthesize cholesterol although 90% of the synthesis occurs in the liver and small intestine.

Lecithin is intimately involved in cholesterol and fat metabolism. It is through the activity of the enzyme, lecithin cholesterol acyl transferase (LCAT), that cholesterol and phospholipids are maintained in balance[35]. The LCAT enzyme is found in the high-density lipoproteins (HDL) or the "good" form of serum cholesterol. As a result, LCAT activity permits dissolution of the cholesterol. In fact, low-density lipoprotein (LDL), the so-called "bad" cholesterol, is rich in cholesterol, whereas HDL is rich in phospholipids. The synthesis of the various transport forms of cholesterol is not likely the result of the presence of phospholipids although dietary phospholipids do affect serum cholesterol levels. Further, a balance of cholesterol, gallic acid (bile) and lecithin is necessary for normal functioning of the gall bladder. Phospholipids in the bile are able to dissolve stone forming cholesterol deposits.

The estimated daily intake of cholesterol is 500 to 600 mg. Cholesterol is decomposed in the liver with 90% being oxidized to gallic acid or excreted as neutral sterols. About 500 to 1500 mg of cholesterol is transported through the bile into the intestine daily. The free cholesterol in the bile is maintained in solution by gallic acid and phospholipids.

Cholesterol may be absorbed at specific sites or receptors[35,48]. This is based on the observation that alternative plant sterols such as sitosterol from soybeans or oryzanol from rice bran oil will inhibit cholesterol absorption[28]

The most common, negative side effect of cholesterol is the formation of cholesterol deposits on the arterial walls damning the flow of blood. The cholesterol deposits restrict blood flow forcing the heart to work harder to supply the blood through the ever-narrowing blood vessels. Eventually, heart disease occurs. The cholesterol content in the coronary arteries of heart attack victims is four times or more that of the average person with normal heart function.

Fats and oils present in our diet are most often referred to as lipids. These are our most concentrated form of energy (Table 7). When consumed and digested, lipids are split into their component parts of fatty acids and glycerol. Lipase enzymes present in saliva, gastric juices, and pancreatic secretions perform the chemical degradation of lipids into fatty acids and glycerol. The degraded lipids may be absorbed as part of the micelles that include cholesterol. Biochemically, saturated fatty acids are known to be cholesterolgenic or promote cholesterol synthesis and polyunsaturated fatty acids promote lowering of cholesterol.

In the intestinal mucosa, the hydrolyzed lipids are recombined inside the subcellular mitochondria present in the mucosa cell protoplasm. The synthesized lipids, essentially adapted to the body since they are synthesized internally, are converted to chylomicrons and very low-density lipoproteins (VLDL) and collected in the thoracic duct.

Phospholipids reach the liver via the portal vein. Digestion is similar as for other lipids. Phospholipase enzymes in the intestine cleave one or both of the fatty acids present in the lecithin. The partially degraded phospholipid is re-synthesized in the intestinal mucosa. The hydrophilic or water soluble, degraded phospholipids are transported to the liver and the lipophilic or fat-soluble fractions are absorbed into the lymph by way of chylomicrons and VLDL.

Table 7   *Energy Content of Dietary Components*

Item	Calories/g	Item	Calories/g
Carbohydrate	4	Protein	4
Fats, oils	9	Lecithin (granular)	7.5

Resorption of phospholipids proceeds in a manner similar to that for cholesterol. Plasma phospholipids, however, consist only of those synthesized in the liver. The synthesis takes place in the endoplasmic reticulum of the cell and the phospholipids leave the liver as components of lipoproteins. The phospholipids participate in the exchange in plasma between HDL and LDL. The most critical step in the exchange is the esterification of cholesterol by the LCAT enzyme (Figure 7). Only the fatty acid in the #2 position of the phospholipid is transferred to the cholesterol. This fatty acid is usually linoleic acid.

A spherical HDL particle results from the combination of a cholesterol ester, a phospholipid and an apoprotein. The apoprotein is a protein specific to the serum transport form of cholesterol. HDL particles also rapidly absorb lecithin from the serum. Phospholipids also are apparently linked with the apoproteins in the HDL and LDL.

3.2 Serum (blood) Lipids (fats)

The nutrients in the foods we eat, the intermediates or breakdown products of metabolism, and the by-products to be excreted are transported in the bloodstream. Fats, oils, lecithin (phospholipids) and cholesterol are present in various forms such as chylomicrons, VLDL, LDL, and HDL. The composition of these carriers of lipids and cholesterol is shown in Table 8.

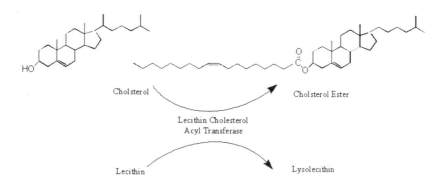

Figure 7. Choline Esterfication

TABLE 8 *Composition of Serum Lipids*

Item	Triglycerides	Cholesterol	Phospholipids	Protein
Chylomicrons	85%–95%	3%–5%	5%–10%	1%–3%
VLDL	60%–70%	10%–15%	10%–15%	10%
LDL	5%–10%	45%	20%–30%	25%
HDL	——	20%	30%	50%

The chylomicrons are formed in the mucosa cells lining the small intestine. Chylomicrons reside in the blood for only a short time (10–60 minutes) emptying their load of triglycerides (lipids) to muscle and fatty tissues. About 20% of the triglycerides, cholesterol and most of the phospholipids are digested or decomposed in the liver.

The triglycerides or fats synthesized in the liver and in the mucosal cells of the small intestine are carried in the blood as VLDL. The rate of VLDL synthesis depends primarily on the free fatty acids present. Reduction of the VLDL begins with hydrolytic splitting of the triglycerides leading to LDL. VLDL remains in the blood for up to 24 hours. It has a half-life of 2 to 4 hours. LDL is also synthesized by other unknown routes.

HDL is synthesized mainly in the liver and contains cholesterol esters. The cholesterol esters are formed by the LCAT enzyme reaction. HDL transfers cholesterol from peripheral tissues to the liver where the cholesterol may be metabolized to gallic acid. A balance of the various types of serum lipids is necessary. Once out of balance (high serum cholesterol and triglycerides, saturated fatty acids, oxidized fatty acids, low HDL, high LDL), injury to the blood vessel walls or deposits may eventually occur resulting in inhibiting blood flow. Supplying lecithin or phospholipids is particularly important to a healthy diet because of their effect on controlling serum lipids. Soybean lecithin, for example, is an excellent source of polyunsaturated fatty acids that are oxidatively stable in addition to the activity of the other individual components present.

CHAPTER 4

Lecithin in Nutrition

4.1 Introduction

The role of lecithin in nutrition is complex. Nearly every cellular and bodily function in some way involves this ubiquitous compound. Much can be traced to specific organs and functions. These are shown graphically in Figure 8. Perhaps as important, lecithin is involved in preventing liver disease and the formation of gallstones.

As discussed, lecithin is involved in cholesterol metabolism and its transport through the blood stream and therefore is important in lowering risks of cardiovascular disease[31,32]. Lecithin is required for synthesis of very-low-density lipoproteins (VLDLs). For this reason, lecithin-deficient diets may begin the process of lipid accumulation in the liver. We also know that lecithin deficiency is connected to the cholinergic nerve transmission diseases[7]. Positive results with lecithin ingestion show that it may play a role in the prevention of diabetes, Parkinson's, Alzheimer's, and Tourettes' syndrome. Important new results from multiple clinical studies have shown that a lecithin deficiency may also play a role in memory impairment. The most recent observations based on scientific evidence have found that lecithin

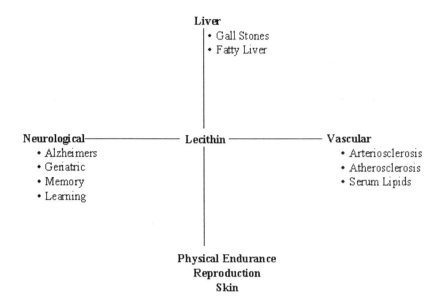

Figure 8. Lecithin in Health

supplementation delays mental aging. The mechanism of action, how and why it works, is unknown.

Contributing to the scientists' and consumers' difficulty in understanding the function of lecithin is that our bodies can synthesize at least part of its own lecithin requirement. It is not a classically "essential" nutrient. However, the study of nutrition has changed from chronic to acute to sub-acute deficiencies. If someone is sub-acutely deficient in lecithin, it is difficult to measure or observe. We do not experience immediate deficiency symptoms. There are no known sub-acute lecithin deficiencies. One cannot help but to conclude that lecithin is not comparable to other essential nutrients that exhibit gross deficiency symptoms. For example, our hair won't fall out, we will not get rickets, and our gums won't swell. This may indicate that only sub-clinical, long-term problems may develop. Perhaps lecithin is only needed for optimum health in a complementary fashion when consumed as part of a total diet. Further, internal synthesis pre-supposes that all substances needed for construction of this compound are present in sufficient quantities at the appropriate times to meet biochemical demands. Some questions about lecithin and its requirement that need answers include: How do we know if our diets are supplying enough of the building blocks of lecithin for adequate synthesis? Can our bodies synthesize enough of the right type at the proper times? Is an external source of this biological nutrient needed to insure adequate supplies for optimum health?

4.2 *Lecithin Is Fundamental To Nutrition*

Lecithin is fundamental to nutrition, being found even in mother's milk (2% of its composition). The infant requires lecithin for cell growth and nerve development, particularly in the formation of the nerve cell insulator, myelin, which surrounds the nerve fiber. Without this insulator, the nerve impulse is dispersed similar to an electric charge from an non-insulated wire when grounded. Lecithin is important in the digestive process for transporting lipids (fats and oils), as an emulsifier in the lymph and blood stream, and it serves as a dietary source of phosphorous, fatty acids and the essential components, choline and inositol. Lecithin protects fats and oils from turning rancid as well as protecting the fat-soluble vitamins from oxidation[33]. Rancid fats are a definite health hazard. Oxidized vitamins are no longer functional vitamins. As an antioxidant, lecithin protects the lipid rich subcellular structures and the integrity of the circulatory system. Lecithin "traps" pro-oxidant metals such as iron and copper and has been added to refined oils to prolong the shelf life, protecting the oil against oxidation or turning rancid. Overall, lecithin is synergistic with tocopherol (vitamin E).

Lecithin is a bioavailable source of choline. Lecithin is a warehouse that can deliver choline upon demand for nerve function and biochemical requirements. It is effectively a timed-release source. It has been found that dietary lecithin supplementation sustains plasma choline at a higher level for a longer period of time than choline chloride when it is taken orally[27,29]. This may be important, as you'll see, for improving physical performance and providing optimum levels of choline to the brain[11].

CHAPTER 5

Associated Diseases

5.1 Cardiovascular Disease (CVD)

Cardiovascular disease (CVD) is the most frequent cause of death in industrialized countries. More than 100 people in the U.S. die each and every hour from heart disease. 51% of adult Americans have blood cholesterol levels of 200mg/dL and higher, a level that is potentially dangerous. Heart disease is so common that it is almost accepted as being normal, and in some cases, a rapid way to "pass on." Fortunately, heart disease and cardiovascular diseases are increasingly being controlled and managed. The principal risk factors are high serum cholesterol, high blood pressure, smoking and the predisposition toward heart attacks. Evidence suggests that lecithin, as a supplement or as a complementary treatment, reduces the risk of CVD by contributing polyunsaturated fatty acids, inhibiting intestinal absorption of cholesterol, increasing the excretion of cholesterol and bile acids, and favorably affecting lipoprotein levels as well as other biochemical events. Several studies have shown lecithin to decrease LDL cholesterol as well as increase HDL cholesterol[34]. Addition of as little as 6 gm lecithin per day to a low-fat, low-cholesterol diet lowered LDL cholesterol by an additional 15 %.

The general types of CVD are arteriosclerosis, atherosclerosis, hyper-proteinemia, and ischemia. Arteriosclerosis is often called "harden-ing of the arteries." This is the most common type of heart condition. It is not an actual heart disease but a disease of the arteries that is caused by fatty deposits containing cholesterol which thicken the ar-terial walls. If it happens in the larger arteries, it brings about symp-toms such as chest pressure pains and angina. An additional thickening of the vascular wall, which further restricts the flow of blood, follows the hardening of the arteries. The major causes are 1) damage to the arterial walls involving lipids, cholesterol and proteins, 2) plaque depo-sition, and 3) diseases of the vascular wall. Oxidized lipids damage or "insult" the lining of the arterial wall. Large quantities of cholesterol are found in these lesions. There is also an increase in phospholipid content but this is believed to be antagonistic to the cholesterol de-posits[16]. In order for LDL cholesterol to cause damage to the arterial wall, it has to be oxidized. If LDL cholesterol is prevented from being oxidized, it does little or no damage. Lipid soluble antioxidants, such as vitamin E, will help overcome this damage. Lecithin demonstrates antioxidant activity[11,33] and is synergistic with vitamin E.

Atherosclerosis, a "silent" disease, is a form of arteriosclerosis that starts with the formation of fatty streaks on the arterial wall and pro-ceeds to the development of complicated insults or lesions (Figure 9). Eventually, restriction of blood flow occurs. Complete restriction is "infarction." Atherosclerosis gets worse as people age. In the U.S., it begins in young people, but in other countries even the elderly show few signs of the disease. Obviously, it is a condition directly related to our diets and how we live. Serum cholesterol, by itself, does not con-stitute an immediate risk of CVD or infarction. There is no scientific cause and effect evidence that high serum cholesterol is a contribu-tory cause of CVD. Statistically, however, the chance for development of atherosclerosis is greater if the cholesterol content of the blood serum is high. Correction of primary imbalances decreases the inci-dence of disease or death from arteriosclerotic cardiovascular disease[35]. More than 30% of Americans in the 45-55 year age group have blood cholesterol levels 240 mg/dL or more. Most studies on CVD have re-

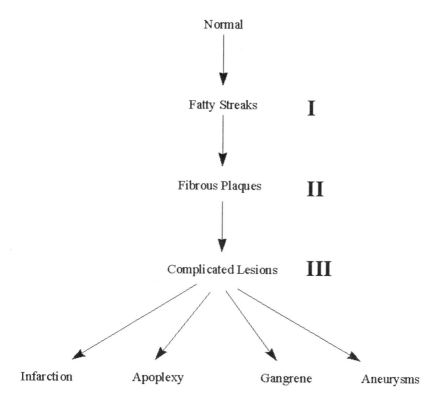

Figure 9. Progression of Atherosclerosis

sulted in statistically derived guidelines. Risk starts at 200 to 250 mg/dl serum cholesterol levels. At these high levels, cholesterol accumulates on the blood vessel wall. As free cholesterol, it is a difficult-to-transport form of cholesterol that may be activated through phospholipid activation of the cholesterol esterase enzyme. Attempts to lower serum cholesterol by dietary restriction results in an increase in cholesterol synthesis in the body. However, if lecithin is added to the diet, the lecithin cholesterol complex is soluble and unwanted cholesterol deposits do not form[10]. The mechanisms behind the cholesterol-lowering properties of lecithin in a high serum cholesterol state, beyond that due to polyunsaturated fatty acid content, are unknown.

Statistically, a high fat diet results in high cholesterol values. Fats differ in their fatty acid composition. Saturated fatty acids have twice the cholesterol-raising power of polyunsaturated fatty acids. Monounsaturated fatty acids are neutral in their cholesterol effect. The fatty acid composition of some of our common fats is listed in Table 9. Most prepared foods are formulated using specialty fats that have been modified by hydrogenation. Hydrogenation results in the formation of both saturated fatty acids and the so-called "trans" or isomeric fatty acids. Trans fatty acids are likely cholesterol forming or cholesterolgenic[36].

Managing the total diet does seem to be one sensible means to control serum cholesterol. Limiting cholesterol-rich foods is a first approach. Eggs, butter, lard, animal fats and shellfish are all high in cholesterol. Consuming polyunsaturated oil containing foods is also advised. Lecithin plus the polyunsaturated oils (e.g. soybean oil, corn oil or olive oil) will help melt the cholesterol away. Basically, the mixture makes it easier to dissolve the cholesterol. In the presence of an oil, the melting point of cholesterol drops to below 32°F. Other dietary recommendations proposed by many involved in cholesterol research are:

1. Addition of dietary fiber (oats, apples, wheat bran, soybeans etc.)

2. Addition of vitamin C with calcium and magnesium

3. Weight management

4. Addition of lecithin to the diet.

A very low serum cholesterol level (<180mg/decl) is also ill advised and can lead to detrimental physiological changes. Cholesterol is even required to maintain red blood cell stability. It is accepted that:

1. HDL is a protective agent

2. High LDL indicates atherogenesis (cholesterol deposits, vascular injury probably present)

3. HDL/LDL ratio is diagnostically significant.

Some guidelines that have been recommended are to have an HDL of more than 55 and an LDL of less than 155. With an HDL of less that 35 and LDL of more than 190 for persons from age 20 to age 50, treatment is believed necessary. Like all recommendations, the absolute numbers are specific to an individual and are subjective.

Lecithin and particularly the choline component of lecithin play a number of other roles in cardiac function. Choline participates in the metabolism of homocysteine, an amino acid that is associated with increased CVD risk[30]. The mechanisms of the atherogenic effects of homocysteine are not known. Choline or lecithin administration can reduce homocysteine levels. "Like folic acid, choline is involved in metabolizing homocysteine and has been shown to be partially effective in lowering homocysteine levels in humans"[37]. Lecithin itself lowers plasma cholesterol and is a key component of various circulatory lipoproteins. Choline is also a key component of plasmalogen, an important phospholipid in the cardiac muscle cell membranes.

5.2 *Vascular Health*

Lecithin is active in preventing vascular disease. Physiologically, lecithin:

1. Prevents vascular diseases associated with fatty deposits.

2. Prevents degenerative arterial diseases.

3. Helps improve the elasticity of blood vessels.

4. Prevents cholesterol from depositing in arterial walls.

Lecithin has specific cholesterol-lowering properties. In animal trials, cholesterol administration to atherosclerotic arteries results in an increase of phospholipid synthesis. The phospholipid detaches the deposited cholesterol and helps to remove the obstruction.

It is important to note that "the anti-atherogenic properties of soy lecithin cannot be attributed solely to the linolenic acid content"[38]. In patients with arteriosclerosis, the concentration of phospholipid com-

TABLE 9 *Fatty Acid Composition of Common Food Oils and Fats*

	Buty	Caproi	Capryl	Capric	Underc	Lauric	Trideca	Myristi	Myrist	Pentad	Pentad	Palmitic	Palmit
Carbon atom (double bonds)	4:0	6:0	8:0	10:0	11:0	12:0	13:0	14:0	14:1	15:0	15:1	16:0	16:1
Babassu		0.4	5.3	5.9		44.2		15.8				8.6	
Butterfat	38	2.3	1.1	2.0	0.1	3.1	0.1	11.7	0.8	1.6		26.2	1.9
Canola Oil												3.9	0.2
Chicken Fat						0.2		1.3	0.2			23.2	6.5
Citrus Seed Oil						0.1		0.5				28.4	0.2
Cocoa Butter								0.1				25.8	0.3
Coconut Oil		0.5	8.0	6.4		48.5		17.6				8.4	
Cohune Oil		0.3	8.7	7.2	0.1	47.3		16.2				7.7	
Corn Oil												12.2	0.1
Cottonseed Oil								0.9				24.7	0.7
Lard				0.1		0.1		1.5		0.2		24.8	3.1
Linseed Oil												4.8	
Murumuru Tallow		0.1	1.3	1.5		46.2		32.4				5.6	0.1
Oat Oil								0.2				17.1	0.5
Olive Oil												13.7	1.2
Palm Oil						0.3		1.1				45.1	0.1
Palm Kernel Oil		0.3	3.9	4.0		49.6		16.0				8.0	
Peanut Oil								0.1				11.6	0.2
Rapeseed Oil								0.1				2.8	0.2
Rice Bran Oil			0.1	0.1		0.4		0.5				16.4	0.3
Safflower Oil								0.1				6.5	
Safflower Oil (high oleic)								0.1				5.5	0.1
Sesame Oil												9.9	0.3
Soybean Oil								0.1				11.0	0.1
Sunflower Oil						0.5		0.2				6.8	0.1
Tallow (beef)				0.1		0.1		3.3	0.2	1.3	0.2	25.5	3.4
Tallow (mutton)				0.2		0.3		5.2	0.3	0.8	0.3	23.6	2.5
Tucum Oil		0.2	2.9	2.3		51.8		22.0				6.8	

Marga	Marga	Stearic	Oleic	Linoleic	Linolen	Nonad	Arachi	Gadolei	Eicosa	Arachi	Beheni	Erucic	Docosa	Lignoceric
17:0	17:1	18:0	18:1	18:2	18:3	19:0	20:0	20:1	20:2	20:4	22:0	22:1	22:2	24:0
		2.9	15.1	1.7			0.1							
0.7	0.2	12.5	28.2	2.9	0.5			0.2		0.1				
		1.9	64.1	18.7	9.2		0.6	1.0			0.2			0.2
0.3	0.1	6.4	41.6	18.9	1.3									
		3.5	23.0	37.8	5.7		0.8							
		34.5	35.3	2.9			1.1							
		2.5	6.5	1.5			0.1							
		3.2	8.3	1.0										
		2.2	27.5	57.0	0.9		0.1							
0.1		2.3	17.6	53.3	0.3		0.1							
0.5	0.3	12.3	45.1	9.9	0.1		0.2	1.3	0.1	.04				
		4.7	19.9	15.9	52.7									
		2.2	8.9	1.5			0.2							
		1.4	33.4	44.8			0.2	2.4						
		2.5	71.1	10.0	0.6		0.9							
		4.7	38.8	9.4	0.3		0.2							
		2.4	13.7	2.0			0.1							
0.1		3.1	46.5	31.4			1.5	1.4	0.1		3.0			1.0
		1.3	23.8	14.6	7.3		0.7	12.1	0.6		0.4	34.8	0.3	1.0
		2.1	43.8	34.0	1.1		0.5	0.4			0.2			0.1
		2.4	13.1	77.7			0.2							
		2.2	79.7	12.0	0.2		0.2							
		5.2	41.2	43.3	0.2									
		4.0	23.4	53.2	7.8		0.3					0.1		
		4.7	18.6	68.2	0.5		0.4							
1.5	0.7	21.6	38.7	2.2	0.6	0.1	0.1				0.4			
2.0	0.5	24.5	33.3	4.0	1.3	0.8					0.4			
		2.3	9.3	2.4										

pounds in the intima or lining of the blood vessel is eight times greater than that in the intima of healthy humans. The explanation is that lecithin formation, particularly phosphatidylcholine, is stimulated mainly in the presence of an adequate supply of polyunsaturated fatty acids. The fats present in the lining of the obstructed vessels are generally composed of saturated or oxidized fatty acids. The stimulated phospholipid synthesis may be the result of efforts by the body to emulsify the deposits. Polyunsaturated phosphatidylcholine lowers LDL cholesterol and likely raises plasma HDL cholesterol. Normal fat metabolism in the blood requires a balance of both lecithin and cholesterol. In a study with patients having hyperlipidemia, those who did not respond to dietary management, when given 3.5g lecithin three times per day before meals for 30 days, showed a 33% decrease in total cholesterol[39]. The LDL cholesterol decreased by 38% while the HDL cholesterol increased by 46%. The triglyceride level also was decreased by 20%. The investigator noted what should be obvious to all, that "lecithin should be administered for the prevention and treatment of arteriosclerosis."

The "stickiness" of blood platelets also responds to lecithin administration. With ingestion of fats or lipids, the tackiness of platelets increases rapidly and substantially but is entirely prevented with 0.2% phospholipids injected into the emulsion. This is also seen for ingestion of aspirin. Aspirin is also known to alleviate vascular disease. Lecithin, however, has none of the potential side-effects associated with aspirin.

Studies have also shown that when lecithin is combined with soy protein, there is a decrease in the LDL and an increase in the HDL. Atherosclerotic manifestations are retarded with resolubilization of the cholesterol upon this dietary regimen.

5.3 Liver Function

Numerous studies have shown that a choline-deficient diet promotes liver cancer or carcinogenesis[40]. The early sign is hepatic lipid accumulation (fatty liver). Phosphatidylcholine is required for synthesis of very low-density lipoproteins (VLDL), the export carrier of triglycerides away from the liver[4]. Fatty liver is followed by cell necrosis, tissue fibrosis, cirrhosis and carcinoma.

During lecithin or choline deficiency, the accumulated liver triglycerides are metabolized to form diacyl glycerides. Plasma membrane protein kinase C (PKC) activity is increased likely contributing to the development of hepatic cancer. Disruption in the phospholipid PKC signaling mechanism may also be involved in other types of cancer such as colon cancer[8]. Trials with lecithin analogs as a cancer treatment are in progress[41].

Lecithin is essential for normal liver function as well. Patients on long-term total parenteral nutrition (TPN), those totally dependent on injection of nutrients, often develop fatty liver infiltration. Lecithin reverses the fatty liver in these patients. Addition of lecithin to the TPN therapy results in an increase of liver density (decreased fat) by 30%.

Lecithin also protects the liver for those who might have high alcohol diets. Animals fed high alcohol diets develop liver cirrhosis without lecithin, but with lecithin supplementation to the animal diet, cirrhosis does not occur. Choline supplementation alone does not provide the protective effect. Those persons with alcohol addiction would, therefore, very likely benefit from taking supplemental lecithin.

5.4 Gall Stones

Cholesterol esters are the transport form of cholesterol formed by the LCAT enzyme system in the HDL. Once transported to the liver, cholesterol is again formed and transported to the gall bladder. In the gall bladder, it is stored together with lecithin resulting in the formation of micelles. The bile acid-cholesterol-lecithin complex is a balanced system. If it goes out of balance, gall stone formation occurs. The gallstones are mainly made up of cholesterol with the most frequent form of gallstone being a cholesterol-bilirubum-calcium stone.

In proper balance of cholesterol, lecithin and bile, dissolution of previously formed gallstones may even occur. It is the lecithin that is largely responsible for dissolution of the stones. Combinations of lecithin with chenodeoxycholic acid, a bile acid, are more effective in dissolving of the stones (0.75gm-chenodeoxycholic acid and 2.25gm lecithin/day). By comparison, the liver supplies about 2 gm phospholipids per day.

5.5 *Nerve and Brain Function*

The blood brain barrier is a selectively permeable tissue with a structure that is interlaced with many membranes. Collectively, the membranes keep harmful substances from the nerve cells. Lecithin is one of the few materials that are able to pass the blood brain barrier. It is believed that lecithin permeability is necessary for the metabolic processes that occur in all cells but also for the constant regeneration of the phospholipid-rich membranes of the brain and for the biosynthesis of phospholipids. Lysolecithin, a partially degraded lecithin, has also been shown to be stored unchanged and intact in the brain. Phosphatidylcholine is also stored intact.

Acetylcholine was previously discussed. A controlled supply of choline is necessary for normal mental behavior. The diseases associated with a malfunction of cholinergic nerve transmission and also involved with acetylcholine are:

- Huntington's chorea

- Friedreich's ataxia

- Tardive dyskinesia: Dystone's syndrome

- Alzheimer's disease

- Gilles de la Tourette's syndrome

Phospholipid addition to the diet has shown some positive clinical improvement in the management of these diseases. Generally, there is considerable improvement for all groups of patients, but the intensity of the disease and the extent of the recovery that has already occurred condition it. In the treatment of these diseases, it can be said that:

- Dietary lecithin is more effective than choline alone.

- De-oiled lecithin is more effective that crude lecithin.

- Improvement in the general health was observed: greater attentiveness, quicker reactions and better orientation were all observed with lecithin.

The distribution of phospholipids in the human brain depends upon age (Table 10). Up to 25% of the dry weight of the brain consists of phospholipids. The brain and spinal cord together contain about 100 grams of phospholipids. The decline with age likely indicates a decline in the synthesis and release of acetylcholine and possible damage to the presynaptic cholinergic receptors. There is less of a decline in choline acyl tranferase (CAT) activity, an enzyme involved in acetylcholine synthesis, when supplemented with large doses of lecithin.

A chronic deficiency of choline may be involved in Alzheimer's disease along with an abnormal processing of amyloid precursor protein. A separate enzyme, called secretase, which is a degradative enzyme in amyloid protein processing, is stimulated by protein kinase C (PKC) but is depressed in Alzheimer's disease. PKC levels are also reduced through chronic choline deficiency[42].

TABLE 10 *Phospholipids in Men's Brain Tissue*

Phospholipid	18-Year-Olds	Gray Matter	White Matter
-Choline	30.3%	39.1%	30.7%
-Ethanolamine	36.2%	40.0%	34.1%
-Inositol	2.6%	—	—
-Serine	17.7%	12.6%	15.7%
Sphingomyelin	13.2%	8.3%	19.5%

Alzheimer's mostly affects cholinergic neurons. These neurons use choline to synthesize acetylcholine. The nerve cells obtain most of their choline from the bloodstream or from choline phospholipids stored in their own membranes[43]. Choline rich diets containing phosphatidylcholine can result in an increase in brain choline and acetylcholine levels[44].

The results of studies on choline and lecithin supplementation alone have not been encouraging in the treatment of Alzheimer's disease, possibly because irreversible changes in the neural pathways may have occurred prior to the addition of supplemental lecithin. The evidence for Alzheimer's disease and amyloid precursor protein may be the result and not the cause of the defect[45]. Tardivedyskinesia, also a defective cholinergic nerve transmission disease, has been successfully treated with phosphatidylcholine[46].

5.6 *Memory*

Age-related memory impairment and disease occurs with everyone. The time of its onset and the degree of impairment vary between individuals. It is also unknown if only short-term or long-term memory is diet or nutrition-related. However, as previously shown, lecithin contains nutrients present in the brain and may be related to memory maintenance.

Our brain acts in computer fashion controlling every bodily function, from the relatively automatic functions of heartbeat and breathing to the more complex functions of memory and thought process. The complex functions of the brain depend upon the presence of neurotransmitters. Acetylcholine is one of the most important neurotransmitters. Lecithin, as noted, is an enhanced form of choline. The choline present in supplemental lecithin will bring about a higher blood level of the substance than that produced by other choline supplements[27]. Perhaps there is an interrelationship between the cholinergic nerve processes and memory. Short-term memory, in particular, is involved with neurotransmitters. While lecithin is not a learning drug, choline administration does result in improved memory as evidenced in learning exercises. Selected positive effects have been observed with memory, cognition, and mobility tests with Parkinson's disease patients. Animal studies also show that lecithin and choline improve memory and learning abilities[47,48]. Rats born to mothers consuming supplemental lecithin possess improved learning[49]. Human studies have suggested a similar improvement of learning and memory[50]. Memory lapses in older adults were significantly fewer (48%) in a lecithin group consuming two tablespoons of granular lecithin per day compared to a control group consuming a placebo.

5.7 *Geriatric Health*

As people age, they lose sharpness in higher level functions of memory and cognition. Both degenerative and retrogressive processes occur. The progressive loss of mental function affects personal productivity, damages self-esteem, and brings distress to aging adults. Defects in memory, depression, nervousness, indigestion, irritability, and circulatory difficulties are among the first signs of the aging process. Methods prescribed to delay the aging process involve:

- A balanced diet adapted to individual need

- Vitamin fortification

- Dietary fiber and minerals

- Exercise.

Cognitive decline with age is individual specific. It normally begins as early as age 50 and is progressive. There are some 30 million residents in the U.S. over age 65, and of these, more than half are experiencing reduced cognitive abilities such as impaired capacity to recall names, numbers, ability to concentrate or recall a word. By the year 2011, the first baby boomers will reach age 65. This generation is the least likely to accept, and will strongly resist, significant declines in memory and cognition.

Memory loss is accompanied by a thinning of the neural network in the brain. Many of the common drugs such as tranquilizers, antidepressants, barbiturates and anticonvulsants damage memory. Much research is underway to conserve the quality of mental function in late adult life. Perhaps most impressive is the very recent information on the affects of lecithin on age related cognitive decline (loss of memory). In tests on senility, lecithin has been found to have a beneficial effect. Patients seem to understand instructions faster and more clearly, and are more cooperative with dietary lecithin supplementation. Regular intake of lecithin supplements improves circulation, perhaps aiding mental function. More rapid clearance of the fats from the blood occurs with lecithin intake along with improved nerve function. Lecithin increases the feeling of well being because it is a source of energy, particularly for the brain, as an alternative to glucose.

Phosphatidylserine, while only a minor constituent of commercial lecithin, has been demonstrated to possess therapeutic activity against age-related memory impairment or loss. It has been shown to delay, and may even reverse, the decline in memory ability as we age. Most studies with phosphatidylserine have been performed with subjects who have had measurable losses in memory, judgment, and other higher mental functions. In these trials, information has been generated by using tests that measure changes in memory, personality, etc. over time in a placebo group and in a treated group. In one study on Alzheimer's patients, improvements were found after PS (phosphatidylserine) administration "on several cognitive measures." "Differences between groups were most apparent among patients with less severe cognitive impairment"[51,52]. Patients with age-associated memory loss who took 100 mg PS three times per day "improved relative to those treated with a placebo"[53]. In some 34 + clinical studies, 14 conducted as double blind trials, together with numerous animal and in-vitro trials, dietary phosphatidylserine enhanced the key measures of lagging brain function[54]. Phosphatidylserine also benefits local nerve networks. The EEG (electro-encephalo graphic) pattern, the HPAA (hyothalamic pituitary-adrenal-axis) pattern related to stress coping in athletes and circadian hormone rhythms, improved memory, learning, concentration, vocabulary skills, mood, alertness, and social ability all improved with the addition of phosphatidylserine to the diet[53,55]. In a clinical blind crossover study, "statistically significant improvements in the phosphatidylserine treated group compared to a placebo were observed both in terms of behavioral and cognitive parameters"[56]. Phosphatidylserine has produced a consistent improvement of symptoms and behavior patterns in conditions of depression. "Phosphatidylserine is the only compound shown to limit and partially reverse age-related memory impairment"[55].

Phosphatidylserine is ubiquitous (present everywhere) in cell membranes and essential to the functions of all cells in the body. It is particularly concentrated in the brain and tissues involved in an assortment of nerve functions including nerve transmitter release and synaptic activity. Phosphatidylserine is present in most common foods but only in very low amounts. Cow's brain is one of the richest sources containing more than 5% phosphatidylserine. Inner organs contain from 1% to 5%. Even in soy lecithin, it is present in only small amounts. As with other phospholipids, phosphatidylserine is not essential since the body can synthesize it. Given orally, phosphatidylserine is rapidly absorbed and, like other phospholipids, can cross the blood brain barrier. In the brain, it likely functions as a component of cell membranes. Supplements were originally available as a bovine brain extract but, with the onset of "mad cow disease," this source is no longer acceptable. Currently, an enzymatically-converted product from soybean lecithin that is high in phosphatidylserine is being produced[51].

As with other phospholipid components, phosphatidylserine shows no danger from long-term intake. It possesses high bioavailability when taken orally. Once consumed, it is evident in the blood in about 30 minutes. Uptake begins in the liver where it passes into the bloodstream and is taken up by the brain. Phosphatidylserine can be enzymatically degraded to phosphatidylethanolamine (PE). PE can in turn be converted to phosphatidylcholine.

Phosphatidylserine is perhaps the most promising brain nutrient discovered in recent years. It is a useful dietary tool for metabolic support of memory, learning, and behavior. Phosphatidylserine isolated from soy lecithin can improve manipulating of information, visual and number recall, and mood compared to control groups receiving a placebo[54]. Dietary supplementation with phosphatidylserine is prudent and advised even though the investigations remain preliminary.

5.8 *Physical Endurance*

Investigations on physical endurance and nutrition have focused on energy and electrolytes. Other factors also play a role in endurance. For example, intense exercise of long duration can and does lower plasma choline levels[58]. This is not surprising since cholinergic nerves also carry signals to muscle fiber. Lecithin and choline supplements prevent the decline in plasma choline and enhance physical performance. In a double blind crossover study, long distance runners improved their times in a 20 mile race from an average of 158.9 minutes on a placebo to 153.7 minutes after choline supplementation[59]. In activities showing plasma choline reductions, choline or lecithin supplementation improves performance.

5.9 *Reproduction*

Choline is recognized as being important for normal development of the brain and the mental capabilities of the fetus and the infant[4,49]. With rats, lecithin addition to the diet results in improved memory of the infant. Surprisingly, the improved memory capability has been shown to extend even to old age. Other likely reproductive effects of lecithin are the synthesis of platelet activating factor (PAF), itself a choline phospholipid. PAF is involved three ways: 1) in implanting of the egg in the uterine wall, 2) in fetal maturation and 3) in inducing of labor[60]. Choline supplementation, including phosphatidylcholine, is even required in infant formulas for balanced nutrition.

Lecithin also plays a role in male fertility. Test tube studies have shown that lecithin has the ability to restore normal structure and movement to abnormal sperm cells and nearly double the acrosomal response.

CHAPTER 6

Lecithin in Your Diet

6.1 *Specifications and types*

The forms of lecithin most widely available are:

- crude or concentrates as liquid products and capsules

- oil-free granules, powders and tablets

- fractionated — phosphatidyl choline and phosphatidylserine

All commercial types currently available are recovered from soybean oil. The quality traits vary as to form supplied. The common traits are:

- Acetone insolubles = AI

- Acid value = AV

- Color = gardener scale

- Fluidity

- Peroxide value = PV

- Moisture

- Microbiological count

The acetone insoluble (AI) number is actually a percentage of the quantity of phospholipids present in a mixture. The minimum AI required by the Code of Federal Regulations for a product to be called "lecithin" is 50%. Capsule and liquid grades of lecithin vary between 50% and 66% AI. Granular and powder forms have an AI greater than 95%. Obviously, the higher the AI, the greater the active constituents and the lesser amounts are required to be consumed. The highest AI supplement available in tablet form is 98%. Specialty lecithins such as phosphatidylcholine or phosphatidylserine vary widely because of diluents being added.

The acid value (AV) is a specification that measures the quality of the crude lecithin. This affects the quantity of oil and the quantity of free fatty acids that may be added to fluidize the crude lecithin. Typical AV's are from 28 to 32. Higher AV's usually occur when the lecithin has been partially degraded due to poor quality soybeans or mishandling of the crude soybean oil.

The color of a liquid lecithin can range from a light straw yellow to almost a strong tea color. A very light color indicates that a hydrogen peroxide bleaching step was most likely used in the preparation of the lecithin. The hydrogen peroxide not only lightens the color but also degrades the fatty acids in the lecithin. A very dark color indicates that process temperatures were too high when drying the wet lecithin after separation from the soybean oil. The dark color results in a loss of phosphatidylcholine, phosphatidylethanolamine and phosphatidylserine. Obviously, very light or dark lecithins are to be avoided to obtain the highest biological activity.

Fluidity is mainly a factor that is important for commercial utilization of liquid lecithin and is of little or no importance to the supplement or capsule market.

The peroxide value (PV) is the only parameter used to determine if hydrogen peroxide was used in the preparation of lecithin or if the product has become partially oxidized. A maximum of 10 PV should be within production limits. Higher values indicate bleach has been used or the product is highly oxidized and is of very questionable quality.

Lecithin in the presence of moisture will undergo microbial spoilage. Moisture contents above 1.0% should be avoided during storage of the lecithin. Most lecithin products are hydroscopic and will attract water from the air. It should be stored in tightly sealed opaque containers for maximum shelf life.

It seems obvious that consumers of lecithin supplements have to rely upon a quality conscious producer and supplier. Many firms are reputable. Choose the supplier having a consistent presence in the marketplace.

6.2   *What Forms of Lecithin Are Available*

Encapsulated lecithins are the easiest form for supplementation. They are a convenient-to-take pre-measured form. However, to prepare capsules, a low AI fluidized product is necessary. The adjustment for fluidity obviously reduces the phospholipid content often to less than 50% of the capsule contents. Granular lecithin forms have greater potency with up to 98% phospholipids being present. The granules have a pleasant "nutty" flavor with a unique, short texture that seems to melt in the mouth when it hydrates during chewing. The granules are easily spread over breakfast cereals, vegetables or even onto desserts. Consumption just before or with meals is advised.

A tabletted form of lecithin has also been produced. The tablets also have a high phospholipid content but with the added convenience associated with capsules. The phospholipid content is the same or greater than that for the granule and powdered forms. Proprietary technology is used in the preparation of this high potency form of lecithin and is distinguished from lecithin tablets prepared by dilution of liquid lecithins with dry powders then tabletted. Tabletted fractionated lecithin are prepared containing pure or enriched forms of the most active lecithins. Phosphatidylcholine and phosphatidylserine tablets and capsules are also available. There are also tabletted-powdered lecithins that use a diluent powder lowering the potency of the final product. Look for the AI value as a primary indication of potency.

Many recipes have been published that allow mixing of the lecithin with other food components. Bakery products (rolls, muffins, breads, waffles, etc.) can be prepared by adding liquid, granule or powdered lecithin equivalent to one tablespoon per serving. Scrambled eggs, soups (particularly, creamed soups), vegetables, meatloaf, pies, and cakes can be prepared and are generally improved functionally with the extra lecithin added to the recipes. Cooking, where there is extreme heat involved such as in deep or skillet frying, destroys the lecithin. The lecithin becomes very dark with a strong noxious burnt odor. Normal cooking does not harm lecithin in more traditional foods.

Drinks are especially adaptable to the incorporation of lecithin. Combinations of one teaspoon of granular lecithin with honey, milk, natural sweeteners and vitamin-mineral mixes make an ideal nutritious drink. Fruit drinks, yogurt and even carbonated drinks are adaptable to including lecithin as a nutrient booster.

CHAPTER 7

A Healthy Diet with Lecithin

Youthful vitality and emotional health are desired by all of us. The capacity of our bodies to function at the highest levels possible depends upon the nutrients we consume. I believe lecithin is one of those nutrients. It assists your body performing a vital role in fat and cholesterol metabolism and has beneficial effects on nerve and brain function. The body can synthesize lecithin. A balanced diet, therefore, must provide either lecithin or the raw material necessary for your body to perform the synthesis of its own lecithin. Supplemental lecithin as phosphatidylcholine and phosphatidylserine or as a mixture circumvents the synthesis, which in some instances is possibly insufficient for optimum performance. In addition to supplements, lecithin-rich foods are to be included in your diet.

The richest natural sources of lecithin and its building blocks are nuts, seeds, whole grains, unrefined oils, organ meats, eggs, butter, and dairy products. However, animal products such as meat, eggs and butter also contain high levels of cholesterol. When we limit our intake of high cholesterol foods, we are actually limiting our lecithin consumption. Supplemental lecithin may be required to offset this deficit.

Many of us have modified our diets to avoid fats at nearly all cost. Combined with refined foods, the typical consumption of lecithin has decreased from over 3 gm/day to less than 1 gm/day. Additionally, both lecithin and vitamin E are removed from vegetable oils during refining. Oils are consequently not a significant source of lecithin. The one gram typically consumed comes from meat and fish, eggs, (a low linoleic acid containing lecithin), and whole grain products. Vegetables and salads contribute almost none. The most favorable lecithin source, most certainly, is from soybeans.

The assumption that 1 gram of lecithin in our diets is sufficient presupposes that our diets are fully balanced and that all metabolic processes are functioning optimally. Even so, it may not be enough. Breathing, metabolism, energy production, energy transport, and nervous function all take place in membranes and mitochondria. These functions are related and dependent on the presence of phospholipids and to the availability of lecithin. Lecithin biosynthesis depends upon an adequate supply of choline which, in turn, depends on methyl donors. Methionine, an amino acid from protein, and choline are closely linked. Lecithin formation is, therefore, partially dependent on protein supply.

There are no risks associated with taking dietary lecithin. It is a biologically active food that is entirely harmless even if taken in large quantities. By taking pure lecithin, it does not require drastic changes in eating habits. The recommended intake of lecithin is 7gm to 10 gm/day (2–3 teaspoonfuls of 3.5gm). For children it is 1–2 teaspoonfuls. Lecithin should be taken regularly over a long period of time. The beneficial effects do not occur immediately or spontaneously, but over a period of 3 months or more. It may be taken with confidence as a preventive or as a health cure without undesirable side effects.

Lecithin is neither a panacea nor a fountain of youth. It is, however, a vital concentrated food whose effects are beneficial and widespread throughout our bodies.

7.1 *Supplemental Lecithin*

Those who previously summarized its nutritional attributes have generally agreed that supplemental lecithin has multiple roles. Together, the physiological and metabolic benefits described by many researchers, producers, writers and scientists may be summarized as:

- Dissolves fats

- Reduces serum cholesterol

- Improves digestibility and fat absorption

- Carries the fat soluble vitamins

- Boosts fat metabolism

- Enhances liver function and kidney health

- Clears cholesterol deposits

- Stimulates nerve function[1,16]

7.2 *Good Health*

The biological roles of lecithin are extensive. This brief overview of recently published information on the many functions of lecithin was aimed at preventing or treating various disease states. A complete review would require a lengthy book, and a Ph.D. in nutritional biochemistry would be necessary for its interpretation. The references listed in the back of this book are for the interested reader who wishes to go deeper into the study of lecithin. For the rest of us, it is sufficient to know that lecithin is a healthy food that is beneficial for the heart and a nutrient for the nerves. The benefits you can experience with continued lecithin supplementation are:

- Improved general health

- Greater attentiveness

- Quicker reaction times

- Improved physical endurance

Once considered a mystical food ingredient, lecithin and its components are actively being researched for their major values in today's nutrition, medicine, and biology. The keys and mechanisms to how it works are just beginning to be understood.

APPENDIX

Lecithin Uses

A.1 *Utilization of Lecithin*

Lecithin has multifunctional properties which are as important to food processors as they are to individual health. Some of these are emulsification, film forming, antioxidation, viscosity reduction, and surface active or surfactant properties (anti-stick). Because of these functional properties, it has uses that range from medicinal to high technology to biochemical. Major quantities of lecithin are utilized in foods, cosmetics, pharmaceuticals, feeds, and miscellaneous applications, and we are now seeing more and more used in nutritional supplements.

The earliest uses of lecithin were for incorporation into chocolate and margarines. Without lecithin addition to chocolate, 25% to 40% more cocoa butter is required for an acceptable chocolate coating. Margarines without lecithin will "weep" during storage and spatter and "pop" when used for frying.

Food and industrial formulators have seen the advantages of lecithin for improving functional properties and to lower costs. Lecithin was adapted for use in bakery, pasta, textiles, paints and even a color copying process[9]. Today, more than 100 million pounds are produced and used annually in the U.S.[17]. Almost all is derived from soybean oil. Animal feeds, particularly that intended for infant animals, take advantage of lecithin's emulsification and nutritional properties. Even farm raised shrimp, trout and salmon have lecithin added to their feeds for improved survival and enhanced growth.

A.2 Lecithin as an Emulsifier (Nature's Surfactant)

The applications of lecithin in foods and non-food products abound[17]. Thousands of products are formulated with lecithin. Just by looking down the grocery isle and reading ingredient labels, lecithin can be found in nearly all formulated foods from cake mixes to margarines. Industrially, lecithin is used in magnetic recording tape, vinyl paints, and as a non-stick coating on conveyor belts and plastic molds. Nearly all applications, whether in food formulations or in paints, take advantage of the "surface-active" properties of nature's surfactant (also called an emulsifier).

Many of the products that utilize lecithin are classified as emulsions. Emulsions are familiar to all of us. Margarines, mayonnaise, and ice cream are commonly cited food examples. Emulsions are mixtures of two insoluble liquids that will separate upon standing. Oil separates from water. Salad dressings rapidly separate into water and oil layers and cream rises to the top from non-homogenized milk. Since we want the mixtures to remain mixed, an additive is needed. The additive is often called an emulsifier. Emulsifiers, then, are ingredients added to stabilize the emulsion, that is, to permit the mixing of two insoluble ingredients.

Emulsifiers are molecules that contain an oil-soluble (lipophilic) portion chemically connected to a water-soluble portion (hydrophilic). These stabilize a dispersed phase (an insoluble product such as oil) in a continuous phase (water). Oil dispersed in water such as dairy cream or whole milk are examples. Naturally present phospholipids and protein stabilize the emulsion. A mayonnaise emulsion contains more than 50% vegetable oil dispersed in water. Egg yolk as a source of lecithin stabilizes this emulsion. Hand soap, dishwashing soaps, and detergents all function based on their emulsifier effect. Each tends to solubilize oil in water.

Lecithin is nature's most widely distributed emulsifier (Figure 10)[10]. It additionally has the unique ability to produce monomolecular layers on the surface of water[11]. Lecithin when used in hand creams and lotions produce an even, thin layer over the surface of the skin producing a subtle feel. Lecithin bar soaps have been developed for prevention of dry or chapped skin. Special lecithins, mainly pure phosphatidylcholine, may be used to encapsulate the oil in moisturizing creams in extremely small droplets or capsules. These extremely small capsules, called liposomes, will penetrate the surface of skin enhancing the effect of a hand or face cream[11].

A.3 *Foods*

The food industry consumes more lecithin than any other industry. Several forms of food grade lecithin are produced that include crude solutions, concentrates, refined liquids, chemically modified liquids and dry granular or powdered products. Quality standards vary widely, along with many specialty products being promoted.

Some of the many food emulsion products containing lecithin are salad dressings, margarines, whipped toppings, ice cream, cake mixes, milk shakes, and coffee creamers. In margarine, lecithin helps the spreadability by softening the fat component. For instantized spray dried products, lecithin assists in the re-dispersion of the dried powders[9]. Instantized dry milk and dry breakfast

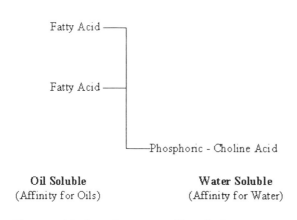

Fatty Acid ———

Fatty Acid ———

———Phosphoric - Choline Acid

Oil Soluble
(Affinity for Oils)

Water Soluble
(Affinity for Water)

Figure 10. Lecithin as an Emulsifier

cocoas are examples. Chocolate is also an emulsion of dry sugar, cocoa and milk solids dispersed in a continuous fat (cocoa butter) phase. About 0.3% to 0.5% of lecithin is added to the chocolate near the end of the 'conching' or emulsifying process to reduce the viscosity of the chocolates for easy pouring into molds or simply coating over the surface of a confectionery piece.

Bakery products are the single largest food use of lecithin. Wheat flour itself naturally contains lecithin[18]. When this lecithin is removed by extraction, the resulting flour does not rise properly or give the desired grain and crumb structure. Additional lecithin improves the texture and shelf life of the finished bakery product.

Overall, lecithin use in foods seldom is above 0.5%[19]. In the price or cost based food industry there has been little attention placed on "healthful" formulations. Cost of goods sold is of primary importance followed by functional performance. Synthetic ingredients that provide greater acceptance and improved functionality are generally chosen over the natural, nutritionally superior lecithin ingredient. Mainstream or mass-market formulated foods cannot be considered as a healthy source of lecithin.

A.4 Cosmetics

Cosmetics can take advantage of the oil-like and film-forming properties of lecithin. A list of the functions of lecithin in cosmetics consists of:

- to form an emulsion

- to improve wetting capabilities

- to assist in dispersing of ingredients

- to act as a synergist to other ingredients

Hand lotions and creams traditionally are promoted as a treatment to overcome dryness, wear, and general decline of the skin[10]. Cosmetics and lotions have been prepared for centuries using proteins and fats to help keep the skin feeling smooth and velvety, while purporting to preserve youthful freshness. These actually work by the simple technique of slowing the loss of water from the surface of the skin. Fats and oils also protect the skin from the ravages of soap, weather, detergents, household chemicals and other irritants. Lecithin, when added to creams and lotions, helps to disperse and spread the fat and other components of lotions such as aromatic compounds and pigments.

Lecithin itself can be used advantageously to prevent dryness of the skin by spreading a film over the skin's surface. Lecithin has "swelling power," meaning that it brings moisture to dry skin along with a desirable re-fatting and re-wetting. Because it is a dispersant, lecithin also assists the penetration of cleaning substances[11]. When combined with natural fats and vitamin E, it protects the skin from attack by oxygen. The unsaturated fatty acids (linoleic and linolenic acid) present in lecithin are also believed to increase the respiratory activity of the skin. Lecithin cosmetics are beneficial in the treatment of skin diseases: eczemas and psoriasis[10].

A formulated lecithin bar similar to hand soap has been produced. This bar contains at least 80% lecithin and may be formulated with other softening and moisturizing components. This all-natural bar is to be used after showering or bathing in the same manner as a soap bar. Even after rinsing and drying, the lecithin bar leaves a thin layer on the skin's surface preventing dry, chapped skin yet having a velvety soft, smooth feel without being waxy or sticky[20]. Traditional soaps are caustic with sodium, potassium and magnesium salts of tallow and palm oil being principle ingredients. Common salt is also often present. These compounds remove the naturally occurring oils from the skin that normally prevent drying or water loss. Lecithin is a natural component of the skin and will neutralize the alkaline or caustic effects of the soap. After showering or bathing is the ideal time to replace oils removed by soaps. The lecithin bar, when moistened, can be simply rubbed over the skin followed by rinsing. The lecithin bar, a source of polyunsaturated fatty acids, may also be fortified with vitamin E, an antioxidant, since both are nutrients for the skin. Additionally, lecithin absorbs ultraviolet (UV) light that is known to adversely affect skin health. Only anecdotal information on the lecithin bar is available at present. Testimonials from users includes descriptions such as "baby-like, youthful soft skin," "makes the wrinkles disappear," "the dry-skin itch disappeared," and "relieves the burning of sunburn."

Recent studies have investigated the effect of topically applied lecithin on serum lipids[21,22]. Initial results surprisingly showed that topically applied phosphatidylcholine reduced the total serum cholesterol and LDL cholesterol, the bad cholesterol, in hypercholesterolemic animals and humans. No doubt further research is needed to determine if this is factual and to identify the mechanism at work. Lecithin has been known to penetrate the skin lending some credibility to this observation. These beneficial effects on serum cholesterol from topical lecithin application have not previously been reported.

A.5 *Pharmaceuticals*

In pharmaceuticals and injectables, lecithin is added as an emulsifying agent to produce an oil in water emulsion. The lecithin may be isolated from natural animal and plant sources. Additional research is ongoing using lecithin in pharmaceuticals. It appears to act beneficially with some drugs. For example, certain anti-inflammatory drugs, classified as nonsteroidal anti-inflammatory drugs (NSAIDS), may cause adverse side effects such as gastrointestinal irritation. They have the well-established ability to cause GI mucosal lesions, perforations and bleeding. In some studies, orally administered lecithin has been shown to be a natural way to protect the stomach lining against these side effects. The lecithin seems to make the walls lining the intestine more "non-wettable," thus protecting it from the corrosive action of the drugs. Lecithin also seems to aid in delivery of some orally administered drugs speeding absorption of the drug.

A.6 *Animal Feeds*

In animal feeds, where we know more about nutrition than we do for human foods, lecithin is incorporated as a physiological and nutritional additive as well as a functional ingredient[23]. Feeds that include lecithin are usually prepared for infant animals: calves, piglets, dogs, cats, trout, shrimp, and salmon. The lecithin improves the digestibility of the animals' high-energy diets primarily through improved dispersion and softening of the fat. Tallow or beef fat becomes as soft as butter with added lecithin. In shrimp feeds, the lecithin improves the utilization of cholesterol, an essential nutrient for shrimp survival and growth. In fact, without the lecithin in aquaculture feeds, shrimp farming would not be economically feasible.

A.7 *Miscellaneous Applications*

Some of the non-food applications of lecithin are magnetic tape production, paints, textiles, greaseless cooking, plastic molding, herbicide dispersions and softening of leather (24). All applications depend upon the film forming and emulsifying functions of lecithin. The active ingredient in greaseless cooking is lecithin, dispersed in alcohol or vegetable oil, with a propellant to allow for spraying. A liquid lecithin-water mix (10:90) may be prepared and used similarly with a pump-spray container. Spray coating the underside of lawn mowers with this mixture prevents grass clippings from sticking. Coating a snow shovel with lecithin prevents the snow from sticking. Barbecue grills are easily cleaned if spray coated with lecithin prior to use.

All of these applications, relying on lecithin's surfactant (non-stick) and emulsifying (combining fats and oil) properties, are but an indication of lecithin's more important and health building biochemical properties and role in human nutrition.

GLOSSARY

Acetylcholine: the chemical transmitter at parasympathetic, some sympathetic, autonomic and somatic motor nerve endings.

Alternative/complementary therapy: providing a choice between treatments.

Anecdotal: a short, entertaining account of some event.

Apoptosis: events leading to death of a cell.

Betaine: an oxidation product of choline metabolism.

Bioavailable: the rate at which a compound enters the blood stream and circulates to the organs.

Bioengineered lipids: fats specifically synthesized to have a desired effect such as non-digestibility or rapid digestibility.

Cardiovascular: refers to all components of the circulatory system including heart, vessels, and arteries.

(K)Cephalin: A phospholipid, phosphatidylethanolamine

Cholesterol: a naturally occurring compound, obtained from plants and animals, which contains partly or completely hydrogenated 17H-cyclopenta-(a)phenanthrene nucleus. It is grouped into the lipids which are fat and fat-like substances.

Choline: a very strong base, a member of the vitamin B complex. It functions in the body to prevent accumulation of fat in the liver and also, as the acetylated derivative acetylcholine, is released at the parasympathetic nerve endings when these nerves are stimulated and thus controls the transmission of impulses across cholinergic synapses.

Cholinesterase: a class of enzymes catalyzing the hydrolysis of acetylcholine.

Cognitive: act or fact of perception; knowledge

CVD: an abbreviation for cardiovascular disease.

Diabetes: diabetes mellitus – chronic disease characterized by excessive sugar in the blood.

Diverticulitis: Inflammation of the diverticular mucosa with attendant complications of peridiverticulitis, phlegmon of the bowel wall, perforation, abscess, and/or peritonitis: obstruction, fistula formation, and bleeding may also be present.

Emulsion: a dispersed system containing at least two immiscible liquid phases, such as water and oil.

Endoplasmic reticulum: a tubular system which courses through the interior of the cell but also appears to communicate with the interstitial space, and its membrane is continuous with the cell membrane.

Essential nutrient: essential food consumed by man to provide energy for growth, maintenance of body functions, and work.

Fiber (dietary): Vegetable fiber, largely indigestible and unabsorbable—mainly a complex mixture of carbohydrate material found in unrefined whole grains, fruits and vegetables.

Food fortification: addition of vitamins, minerals for "enriched" consumption.

Food pyramid: hierarchal chart of foods recommended to be consumed for nutritional health. Contains carbohydrates, fats, and proteins in natural presence. Lists grains, fruits, vegetables, meats, dairy.

GI: gastrointestinal—relating to stomach and intestines

Glycerol = glycerin: a sweet, oily liquid obtained from fats and oils; the simplest trihydric alcohol.

Hematopoiesis: the process of formation and development of blood cells.

Homocysteine: a degradation product of the amino acid, methionine.

Hydrate: a combination with water; chemically, a binding with water.

Inositol: $C_6H_6(OH)_6$, a vitamin of the B complex that is essential for growth of mice and yeast; found in plants often as the hexaphosphate, phytic acid.

Iodine value: a determination of the degree of unsaturation in a fat or oil. A high iodine value, eg 130, indicates a high content of unsaturated fatty acids.

Ischemia: obstruction of the blood supply.

Kinase: an enzyme catalyzing the transfer of phosphate groups.

LCAT: lecithin cholesterol acyl transferase—an enzyme that reversibly transfers a fatty acid from lecithin to cholesterol forming a cholesterol ester.

Linoleic acid: a polyunsaturated fatty acid that is a liquid, $C_{18}H_{32}O_2$, found in soybean oil, linseed oil and other vegetable oils.

Lipids: any of a group of organic substances, including fats, sterols, and waxes, insoluble in water but able to be metabolized.

Lipoidal: a term meaning resembles fat; an older term for lipids.

Methionine: an essential amino acid containing sulfur and methyl groups. May be used in warding off or treating certain diseases of the liver.

Methyl donor: carbon radical (CH3) chemical donor; Methyl donors are methionine and choline.

Micelle: a water soluble or dispersible aggregate of microscopic size.

Microsome: one of the minute granules present in the protoplasm of animal and plant cells.

Myocardial infarction = MI: Ischemic myocardial necrosis usually resulting from abrupt reduction in coronary blood flow to a segment of myocardium (heart). Insufficient arterial or venous blood supply to the heart.

Neural messages: messages transferred from one nerve cell to the next.

Non-caloric fats: compounds having fat or oil characteristics but are non-digestible.

Omega 3 fatty acids: long chain length fatty acids with unsaturation three carbons from the methyl end.

Organ meats: meat derived from liver, kidney, intestine or pancreas.

Parenteral: intravenous injection other than through the gastrointestinal tract.

Phosphatide: general chemical name for lecithin.

Phospholipase A: an enzyme catalyzing the hydrolysis of a fatty acid from the lecithin molecule.

Phospholipids: a lipid (lecithin) containing phosphorus.

PC: phosphatidylcholine

PE: phosphatidylethanolamine

PI: phosphatidylinositol

PS: phosphatidylserine

Phytic acid: the phosphoric acid derivative of inositol.

Placebo: a pill or liquid with little or no therapeutic value given merely to please the patient, or given as a control in experiments testing the effectiveness of a drug.

Plasmalogen: general term for phospholipids containing an ether or aldehyde groups.

Prepared foods: foods ready for consumption with a minimum of preparation.

Protein: class of complex chemical compounds which contain carbon, hydrogen, nitrogen, oxygen, and sulfur; involved in forming structures, hormones, enzymes and all functions of living matter; hydrolysis yields various amino acids.

Red meat: a general classification of meats from beef, swine ,deer and other ruminants

Serum cholesterol: cholesterol present in the fluid portion of the blood.

Soy food: foods prepared from soybeans or soybean products such as tofu or soymilk.

Spingomyelin: a group of phospholipids found in the brain, spinal cord, etc having a long chain fatty acid amide present.

Subcellular: less than or contained within the cell.

Supplement: additions to diet made up of vitamins, minerals, and essential dietary nutrients.

Surfactant: compounds referred to as wetting agents, solubilizing agents and emulsifying agents.

Vascular disease: diseases of the blood vessels, heart and circulatory system.

REFERENCES

1. USDA Nationwide Food Consumption Survey. Washington, DC., United States Department of Agriculture, 1979.
2. USDA. Continuing Survey of Food Intakes by Individuals. Washington, DC., United States Department of Agriculture, 1992.
3. Wade, Carlson, *Lecithin Book*. Keats Pub. Inc. New Canaan, Connecticut, 1980
4. Zeisel, S.H., Choline, p.449-458 in *Modern Nutrition in Health and Disease*. 8th ed. M.E. Shils, J.A. Olsen, M. Shike, ed. Lea and Febiger. Phila., 1994.
5. Messina, M., and V. Messina, and K.D.R. Setchell. The Simple Soybean and Your Health. Avery Pub. Group, Garden City Park, NY.,1994
6. Davis, A. *Lets Eat Right to Keep Fit*. Penguin Pub. New York, 1970.
7. Yates, J., Lecithin works wonders. Prevention 32: 55-59., Feb. 1980.
8. Carty, D. J., S.H. Zeisel and J.J. Jolitz. *Lecithin and Choline.*, Central Soya Co. Fort Wayne, IN., 1996.
9. Szuhaj B. and G. List. *Lecithins*. American Oil Chemists' Society monograph 12. Champaign, IL., 1985.
10. Schafer, W. and V. Wywiol. *Lecithin—The Unrivaled Nutrient*. Stern-Chemie. Hamburg, FRG. 1988.
11. Ceve, G. and F. Pltanf, eds. *Phospholipids: Characterization, Metabolism, and Novel Biological Applications*. American Oil Chemists Society Press. Champaign, IL. 1995.
12. Stampfer, M.J., M.R. Malinow, W.C. Willett, et. Al. A prospective study of plasma homocyst(e)ine and risk of myocardial infarction in U.S. physicians. JAMA 268: 877-881. 1992.

13. Selhub, J. P.F. Jacques, A.G. Bostom, et. Al. Association between plasma homocysteine concentrations and extracranial carotid-artery stenosis. N. Engl. J. Med. 332: 286-291. 1995.
14. Arnesen, E., H. Retsum, K.H. Bonaa, et. al. Serum total homocysteine and coronary heart disease. Intnl. J. Epidemics. 24: 704-709. 1995.
15. Gross, R.W. Accelerated phospholipid catabolism as a mediator of ischemic injury: enzymes and molecular conformations. Presented at *Choline Phospholipids: Molecular Mechanisms for Human Diseases*. Univ. of North Carolina / Amer. Inst. Of Nutrition. San Diego, CA. 1992.
16. Szuhaj, B.F. ed. *Lecithins: Sources, Manufacture and Uses*. American Oil Chemists Society. Champaign, IL. 1989.
17. Sipos, E.F. and B.F. Szuhaj. *Lecithins in Bailey's Industrial Oil and Fat Products*. John Wiley and Sons, Inc. New York. 1996.
18. Orthoefer, F.T. Lecithin: a natural emulsifier. Presented at American Oil Chemists' Society annual meeting. San Antonio, TX. 1995.
19. Orthoefer, F.T. and S.U.Gurkin. Lecithin—the universal ingredient. Intl. Food Marketing and Technology. 6:6. 1992.
20. Orthoefer, F.T. U.S., Patent Application, Nutricor. 1996.
21. Hsia, S.L., J.L. He, Y. Nie, K. Fong and C. Milikowski. The hyposcholesterolemic and antiatherogenic effects of topically applied phosphatidylcholine in rabbits with heritable hypercholesterolemia. Artery 22: 1-23. 1996.
22. Hsia, S.L., J.L. He, M. Mandel and C.W. Froelich. Lowering serum cholesterol by topical treatment with soy phophatidylcholine. Presented at 7th International Congress on Phospholipids. Brussels, Belgium. Sept. 1996.
23. Orthoefer, F.T. , S.U. Gurkin and J.D. Fisk. The use of soybean lecithin in aquaculture. Ch. 10 in *Nutrition and Utilization Technology in Aquaculture*. C. Lim and D. Sessa, eds. American Oil Chemists Press. Champaign, IL 1995.
24. Orthoefer, F.T. and J. Schmidt. Non-food uses of lecithin Ch. 9 in *Lecithins*. B. Szuhaj and G. List, American Oil Chemists' Society monograph 12. Champaign, IL 1985.
25. Zeisel, S. Choline Phospholipids: signal transduction and carcinogenesis. FASEB J. 7: 551-557, 1993.
26. Canty, D.J. and S.H. Zeisel. Lecithin and choline in human health and disease. Nutr. Rev. 52: 327-329. 1994.

27. Hirsch, M.J., J.H. Growdon, and R.J. Wurtman. Relations between dietary choline or lecithin intake, serum choline levels and various metabolic indices. Metabolism 27: 953-960. 1978.

28. Code of Federal Regulations. 21 CFR para. 182, 184. Office of the Federal Register. U.S. Govt. Printing Office. Washington DC. 1995.

29. Wurtman, R.J., M.J. Hirsch and J.H. Growdon. Lecithin consumption raises serum-free-choline levels. Lancet July 9, 68-69. 1977.

30. Orthoefer, F.T. Rice bran oil: healthy lipid source. Food Technology 50 (12):62-64. 1996.

31. Malinow, M.R. Hyperhomocyst(e)inemia: a common and reversible risk factor for occlusive atherosclerosis. Circulation 81: 2004-2006. 1990.

32. O'Brien, B.C. and V.G. Andrews. Influence of dietary egg and soybean phospholipids and triacylglycerols on human serum lipoproteins. Lipids 28: 7-12.

33. Sugino, H., M. Ishikawa, et. al. 1997. Antioxidant activity of egg yolk phospholipids. J. Agric Food Chem. 45, 551-554.

34. Childs, M.T., J.A. Bowlin, et. al. 1981. The contesting effects of dietary soya lecithin product and corn oil on lipoprotein lipids in normolipidemic and familial hypercholesterolemic subjects. Atherosclerosis 38, 217-222.

35. Frick, M.H., O.Elo, et.al. Helsinki heart study, primary prevention trial with gemfibrozil in middle-aged men with dyslipidemia. Safety of treatment, changes in risk factors, and incidence of coronary heart disease. N. Eng. J. Med. 317, 1237-1245. 1987.

36. Mensink, R.P. and M.B. Katan. N. England J. Med. 325: 439. 1990.

37. McCully, K.S. Homocysteine and vascular disease: role for folate, choline, and lipoprotein in homocysteine metabolism. Presented at 7th International Congress on Phospholipids. Brussels, Belgium. Sept. 1996.

38. Wilson, T.A., C. Meservey and R. J. Nicolosi. 1997. The hyposcholesterolemic and anti-atherogenic effects of soy lecithin in hypercholemic monkeys and hamsters: beyond linoleate. J. Nutr. Biochem. (in press).

39. Wojeieki, J., A.Pawlik, et.al. 1995. Clinical evaluation of lecithin as a lipid-lowering agent. Phytotherapy Res. 9,597-599.

40. Locker, J., T.V. Reddy and B. Lombardi. DNA methylation and hepatocarcinogenesis in rats fed a choline devoid diet. Carcinogenesis 7: 1309-1312. 1986.
41. Houlihan, W.J., M. Loh Meyer, P. Workman and S.H. Cheon. Phospholipid antitumor agents. Med. Res. Rev. 15: 157-223. 1995.
42. Gillespie, S.L., T.E. Golde, and S.G. Younkin. Secretory processing of Alzheimer amyloid B/A4 protein precursor is increased by protein phosphoylation. Biochem. Biophys. Res. Com. 187: 1285-1290. 1992.
43. Wurtman, R.J. Phosphatidylcholine in neurologic disorders. *Choline Phospholipids: Molecular Mechanisms for Human Diseases*. Satellite conference, Univ. of North Carolina / Amer. Inst. Of Nutrition. San Diego CA. 1992.
44. Cohen, E.L. and R. J. Wurtman. Brain acetylcholine: control by dietary choline. Science 191: 561-562. 1976.
45. Zeisel, S.H. Lecithin in health and human nutrition p225-236 in *Lecithin: Sources, Manufacture and Uses*. B. Szuhaj, ed. American Oil Chemists' Society. Champaign, IL. 1989.
46. Greenberg, A.J., J.D. Wojcik, and J.H. Growden. Lecithin for the treatment of Tardive dyskinesia. P205-303. In *Nutrition and the Brain: Choline and Lecithin in Brain Disorders*. A. Barbeau, J.H. Growden, and R.J. Wurtman, eds. Raven Press. New York. 1979.
47. Bartus, R.T., R.L. Dean, A.J. Goas, and A.S. Lippas. Age related changes in passive avoidance retention: modulation with dietary choline. Science 209: 301-303. 1980.
48. Izaki, Y., M. Hashimot, J. Arita, M. Iriki and H. Hibno. Intraperitoneal injection of 1-oleoyl-2-docosaheenoil phosphatidylcholine enhances discriminatory shock avoidance learning in rats. Neurosci, Letters 167: 171-174. 1994.
49. Meek, W.H. Choline and development of brain memory functions across the lifespan. Presented at the 7th International Congress on Phospholipids. Brussels, Belgium Sept. 1996.
50. Sitaram, M., H. Weingartner, and J. C. Gillin. Human serial learning: enhancement with choline and impairment with scopolamine. Science 201:2274-276. 1978.
51. Crook, T., W. Petrie, et. al. 1992. Effects of phosphatidylserine in Alzheimer's disease Psychopharmocol. Bull 28 (1), 61-66
52. Crook, T.H. 1991. Effects of phosphatidylserine in age-associated memory impairment. Neurol. 41,644-649.

53. Crook, T.H. et al. Effects of phosphatidylserine in age-associated memory impairment. Neurology 41: 644. 1991.

54. Kidd, P.M. Phosphatidylocrine, cell membrane nutrient. Rationale for its benefit against cognitive decline. Abst. American Oil Chemists' Society annual meeting. May 11-14. Seattle WA 1997.

55. Crook, T.H. Effects of phosphotidylserine on age-related learning and memory defects. Abst. American Oil Chemists' Society annual meeting. May 11-14. Seattle, WA. 1997.

56. Cenacchi, T., T. Bertoldin, et. al. 1993. Cognitive decline in the elderly: a double-blind, placebo-controlled multicenter study on efficacy of phosphatidylserine administration. Aging 5 (2), 123-133.

57. Schneider, M. Soybean phosphatidylserine manufacturing process and safety evaluations. Abst. American Oil Chemists' Society annual meeting. May 11-14. Seattle, WA. 1997.

58. Conlay, L.A., R.J. Wurtman, et. al. Decreased plasma choline concentration in marathon runners. N. Eng. J. Med. 315: 892. 1986.

59. Sandage, B.W., R.N. Sabounjan, et. al. Choline citrates may enhance athletic performance. Physiologist. 1992; 35:236a.

60. Johnston, J.M. The role of platelet-activation factor (PAF) in reproductive biology. Presented at: Choline Phospholipids: Molecular Mechanisms for Human Diseases. Univ. of North Carolina / Amer. Inst. Of Nutrition. San Diego, CA April 3, 1992.

61. King, J.C. 1996. Recommended daily intake for choline and choline phospholipids. Presented at American Oil Chemists' Society annual meeting. Indianapolis, IN. May 1.